Workbook of Solutions and Dosage of Drugs

INCLUDING MATHEMATICS

Workbook of Solutions and Dosage of Drugs

INCLUDING MATHEMATICS

THORA M. VERVOREN, R.Ph., B.S.

Director, Pharmacy Service, Columbia Hospital,
Milwaukee, Wisconsin

JOAN E. OPPENEER, R.N., M.S.N.

Professor Emerita, University of Wisconsin-Milwaukee
School of Nursing, Milwaukee, Wisconsin

TWELFTH EDITION

The C. V. Mosby Company

ST. LOUIS   TORONTO   1983

MOSBY

A TRADITION OF PUBLISHING EXCELLENCE

Editor: Julie Cardamon
Assistant editor: Bess Arends
Manuscript editor: Patricia J. Milstein
Design: Suzanne Oberholtzer
Production: Judy Bamert

TWELFTH EDITION

Printed in the United States of America

International Standard Book Number 0-8016-5228-6

The C.V. Mosby Company
11830 Westline Industrial Drive, St. Louis, Missouri 63146

TS/VH/VH 9 8 7 6 5 4 3 2 1 03/C/330

Preface

This workbook is primarily designed for students in nursing and is a useful resource for nurses returning to practice. Pharmacy students and pharmacy technicians will also find the workbook a valuable learning resource. The purpose of the book is to provide learning activities that will assist the student to develop knowledge and skills necessary to safely participate in components of patient care related to drug therapy.

The workbook has been developed to be used as a text for a course in drugs and solutions, as a supplement for a course in pharmacology, and as a self-study program for health care professionals. The objectives that precede each chapter, the practical problems related to current drug therapy, and the tests that can be self-administered make the book an adaptable resource.

The concise "Review of Mathematics" that precedes the sections related to pharmaceutical calculations can be completed independently and followed with the survey test. "Systems of Measurement" provides basic information on the apothecaries' and metric systems, conversion from one system to another, and the conversion of Celsius and Fahrenheit temperature measurement. "Calculation of Dosage" is based on practical drug problems encountered in clinical practice. All problems of external, oral, parenteral, and pediatric dosage calculations relate to actual health care situations. This approach assists the student to more readily relate theory to practice. Answers to problems and a comprehensive examination are located in the Appendix.

We express our appreciation to faculty and students for their suggestions that have been incorporated into this revision, and to Paula Meyer for typing the manuscript.

Thora M. Vervoren
Joan E. Oppeneer

To Students

This book is designed for guided or independent study. Objectives preceding each chapter will guide you in determining your achievements. Practical drug problems that follow each chapter may be worked in the spaces provided and may be used as a future reference. Answers to the drug problems are located in the Appendix and may be used in evaluating your work.

Contents

PART 1

REVIEW OF MATHEMATICS

- Arabic and Roman Number Systems
- Fractions and Ratio
- Decimals
- Percentage and Proportion

CHAPTER 1

Arabic and Roman Number Systems

OBJECTIVES

At the completion of this chapter, the student will:

- differentiate the Arabic system from the Roman system of numbers
- convert Arabic numerals to Roman numerals
- convert Roman numerals to Arabic numerals

The history of the system of numbers is assumed to go back in time before recorded history. Each country had its own system, and as communications and exchange of goods between peoples increased, the need for a common system of numbers increased. The system of numbers with which we are familiar is derived from the early systems of the Arabians, Hindus, Babylonians, Assyrians, Egyptians, and tribes unnamed in history.

The early system of notation was largely a system of counting. This type of notation was similar to our whole number. In time another kind of notation made its appearance. It was used in designating a part of a whole and was called a broken number or fraction. Earliest history of a broken number or fraction comes from the Egyptians and Babylonians. As the system of notation developed, the Greeks followed the Egyptian system of fractions and the Romans the Babylonian system of fractions. By the end of the sixteenth century the surviving systems of numbers were the Arabic and Roman.

THE ARABIC SYSTEM OF NOTATION

Arabic numerals are 1, 2, 3, 4, 5, 6, 7, 8, 9, 0.

The Arabic system has surpassed and supplanted all other systems because it is simple and versatile. A numeral expresses a number and a combination of numerals expresses other numbers. Each numeral has a place value beginning from right to left. In a number such as 245, 5 is in the one's place expressing 5 ones; 4 is in the ten's place expressing 4 tens; 2 is in the hundred's place expressing 2 hundreds. Successive numerals occupy a place whose value is ten times as much as the preceding one.

Another advantage of the Arabic system is that it is readily adapted to use with broken numbers or fractions. This is indicated by the numerals to the right of one's place. The separation of whole numbers, a broken number, or fraction is indicated by a symbol. The most common is the decimal point.

The four basic processes of computation—addition, subtraction, multiplication, and division—can be carried out in the Arabic system.

THE ROMAN SYSTEM OF NOTATION

The Romans used letters to designate numbers. This restricts the system's usefulness, since there is no way to indicate processes in arithmetic such as division or multiplication. Roman numerals are sometimes used on dials of clocks and watches, for dates, especially on public buildings, and to head chapters in books. Roman numerals are used in the apothecaries' system of measures in writing prescriptions and dosage of drugs.

Basic Roman numerals are expressed by seven capital letters as follows:

Roman numeral	Arabic equivalent
I	1
V	5
X	10
L	50
C	100
D	500
M	1000

$\overline{\text{D}}$ = 5000, and $\overline{\text{M}}$ = 10,000, but these are seldom used.

Roman numerals also may be expressed in lower case letters.

When Roman numerals are used to write dosage of drugs and prescriptions, the numerals are expressed in lower case letters. The most commonly used lower case Roman numerals are as follows:

Roman numeral	Arabic equivalent
i	1
v	5
x	10
l	50

A combination of Roman numerals expresses other numbers.

Rule I—addition indicated

1. When a numeral of lesser value follows one of greater value.

2. When numerals of the same value are repeated in sequence. However, numerals are never repeated more than three times in a sequence.

EXAMPLES:

1. VI = 5 + 1, or 6
   XV = 10 + 5, or 15

2. II = 1 + 1, or 2
   III = 1 + 1 + 1, or 3
   XXX = 10 + 10 + 10, or 30

Rule II—subtraction indicated

1. When a numeral of lesser value precedes one of greater value.

2. When a numeral of lesser value is placed between two of greater value, the numeral of lesser value is subtracted from the numeral following the one of lesser value.

EXAMPLES:

1. IV = 5 − 1, or 4
   IX = 10 − 1, or 9
   XL = 50 − 10, or 40

2. XIV = 10 + 5 − 1, or 14
   XXIX = 10 + 10 + 10 − 1, or 29
   MCMLXXXIII = 1000 + 1000 − 100 + 50 + 10 + 10 + 10 + 3 or 1983

PROBLEMS

Name ______________________

Date ______________________

ARABIC AND ROMAN NUMBER SYSTEMS

1. Write the following Arabic numerals as basic Roman numerals:

56	______	448	______
100	______	60	______
40	______	210	______
30	______	919	______
1550	______	27	______
656	______	85	______
504	______	99	______
1985	______	259	______

2. Write the following Roman numerals as Arabic numerals:

CCL	______	DCC	______
CDLV	______	DCL	______
MCMLXXV	______	DCX	______
XCIV	______	MM	______
CX	______	IV	______
XXIX	______	LVI	______
XVII	______	IX	______
XXXIII	______	XI	______
L	______	MXL	______
VC	______	LXXXIX	______

3. Write the following Arabic numerals as lower case Roman numerals:

6	______	3	______
14	______	51	______
22	______	7	______
19	______	18	______
1061	______	155	______

4. Write the following lower case Roman numerals in Arabic numerals:

ix	______	xl	______
xxiv	______	xii	______
lxv	______	xxix	______
iv	______	lxxi	______
cxli	______	xxxv	______

CHAPTER 2

Fractions and Ratio

OBJECTIVES

At the completion of this chapter, the student will:

- identify various kinds of fractions
- change the form of fractions
- compute fraction problems
- compute ratio problems

A fraction is a number that indicates division. In a simple form it expresses one or more parts into which a unit is divided.

EXAMPLES:

$\frac{1}{3}$ is one part of a unit that is divided into three equal parts.

$\frac{2}{7}$ is two parts of a unit that is divided into seven equal parts.

$\frac{3}{8}$ is three parts of a unit that is divided into eight equal parts.

The **numerator** is the dividend, or the number above the line. It tells how many parts of the divided unit are taken.

The **denominator** is the divisor, or number below the line. It tells into how many parts the unit is divided.

The numerator and denominator are called the **terms** of a fraction.

EXAMPLE: $\frac{2}{5}$ 2 is the numerator; 5 is the denominator. 2 and 5 are the terms.

As the denominator of a fraction increases, the value decreases if the numerator remains the same.

$$\frac{1}{2}, \frac{1}{3}, \frac{1}{5}, \frac{1}{10}, \frac{1}{20}$$

The fractions in this series are from greater to lesser value. It is possible to add, subtract, multiply, and divide fractions in the same manner as whole numbers.

KINDS OF FRACTIONS

1. A **proper fraction,** often called a simple or common fraction, is a fraction in which the numerator is smaller than the denominator. It is less than one unit.

EXAMPLES: $\frac{1}{4}$, $\frac{7}{9}$, $\frac{2}{3}$

2. An **improper fraction** is a fraction in which the numerator is equal to or greater than the denominator. It is equal to one unit or more than one unit.

EXAMPLES: $\frac{3}{2}$, $\frac{11}{3}$, $\frac{8}{8}$

3. A **mixed number** is a whole number and a fraction. Its value is always more than one unit.

EXAMPLES: $2\frac{1}{9}$, $8\frac{6}{7}$

4. A **complex fraction** is a fraction in which the numerator or the denominator is a fraction, or the numerator and denominator are both fractions.

EXAMPLES: $\dfrac{5}{\frac{1}{2}}$, $\dfrac{\frac{1}{2}}{5}$, $\dfrac{\frac{2}{3}}{\frac{5}{6}}$

In these fractions 5, $\frac{1}{2}$, and $\frac{2}{3}$ are the numerators; $\frac{1}{2}$, 5, and $\frac{5}{6}$ are the denominators.

LIKE AND UNLIKE FRACTIONS

Fractions whose denominators are alike, such as $\frac{2}{7}$, $\frac{3}{7}$, and $\frac{5}{7}$, are called **like fractions.**

Fractions whose denominators are unlike, such as $\frac{1}{3}$, $\frac{1}{4}$, and $\frac{2}{5}$, are called **unlike fractions.**

Like fractions can be added, subtracted, multiplied, and divided.

Unlike fractions can be multiplied and divided. Therefore when addition or subtraction of unlike fractions is indicated, it becomes necessary to change the unlike fractions to like fractions. The change results in a new fraction, different in form but equal to the original fraction, which is called an equivalent fraction.

EQUIVALENT FRACTIONS

The equivalency of fractions is based on a fundamental principle in computing with fractions: *Multiplying or dividing both terms of a fraction by the same number does not change its value.*

Computing with fractions depends on this principle. Multiplying or dividing both terms of a fraction by the same number results in another fraction of the same value and is called an **equivalent fraction.**

EXAMPLES:

1. Multiply both terms of $\frac{3}{4}$ by 2; by 4:

$$\frac{3 \times 2}{4 \times 2} = \frac{6}{8} \qquad \frac{3 \times 4}{4 \times 4} = \frac{12}{16}$$

The resulting fractions $\frac{6}{8}$ and $\frac{12}{16}$ are equal to $\frac{3}{4}$ and to each other.

When both terms of a fraction are multiplied by the same number, the terms of the new fraction are **larger** than the terms of the original fraction.

2. Divide both terms of the fraction $^{12}/_{16}$ by 4; $^{6}/_{8}$ by 2.

$$\frac{12 \div 4}{16 \div 4} = \frac{3}{4} \qquad \frac{6 \div 2}{8 \div 2} = \frac{3}{4}$$

The resulting fraction $^{3}/_{4}$ is equal to $^{12}/_{16}$ and $^{6}/_{8}$; therefore $^{12}/_{16}$ and $^{6}/_{8}$ are equal to each other.

When both terms of a fraction are divided by the same number, the terms of the new fraction are **smaller** than the terms of the original fraction. A fraction changed to its smallest terms simplifies computing by reducing the possibility of errors and by saving time. The process of changing the terms of a fraction to smaller terms is known as *reducing a fraction to its lowest terms.*

CONVERSION OF UNLIKE FRACTIONS

There are several methods by which two or more unlike fractions can be converted to like fractions. One method consists of the following two steps: (1) find the lowest multiple that will be common to the denominators of the fractions under consideration, and (2) convert each original fraction to an equivalent fraction having the lowest common multiple as the denominators.

Step I

To find the lowest multiple that will be common to the denominators of unlike fractions, divide all the numbers in the denominators of the fractions by a factor that is common to two or more of them and that will divide into them evenly; continue until no two numbers in the quotient are divisible by the same number. Multiplying all the divisors and the remaining numbers greater than one results in the least common multiple (LCM).

EXAMPLE: In the fractions $^{2}/_{3}$, $^{3}/_{5}$, $^{5}/_{6}$, and $^{1}/_{12}$ the LCM of the denominators is 60. Therefore 60 will be the denominator of the equivalent fractions.

$$\begin{array}{r|l} 3 & 3 - 5 - 6 - 12 \\ \hline 2 & 1 - 5 - 2 - 4 \\ \hline & 1 - 5 - 1 - 2 \end{array}$$

$$3 \times 2 \times 5 \times 2 = 60 \text{ (LCM)}$$

Step II

To obtain the numerators of the equivalent fractions, multiply each original fraction by the LCM obtained in Step I. Place the product over the LCM.

EXAMPLE: Change $^{2}/_{3}$, $^{3}/_{5}$, $^{5}/_{6}$, and $^{1}/_{12}$ to equivalent fractions with a denominator of 60.

$$\frac{2}{\cancel{3}} \times \overset{20}{\cancel{60}} = 40 \qquad \frac{3}{5} \times \overset{12}{\cancel{60}} = 36 \qquad \frac{5}{\cancel{6}} \times \overset{10}{\cancel{60}} = 50 \qquad \frac{1}{\cancel{12}} \times \overset{5}{\cancel{60}} = 5$$

Placing the product over the denominator gives the equivalent fraction.

$$\frac{2}{3} = \frac{40}{60} \qquad \frac{3}{5} = \frac{36}{60} \qquad \frac{5}{6} = \frac{50}{60} \qquad \frac{1}{12} = \frac{5}{60}$$

To prove, reduce the equivalent fraction to its lowest terms. The result should be the original fraction.

In some fractions the product of the denominators is the LCM, and sometimes the larger denominator of two or more fractions contain the smaller denominator two or more times. These can be recognized easily; therefore Step I would be unnecessary.

EXAMPLES:

1. $^3/_4$ and $^1/_5$
2. $^1/_6$ and $^5/_{18}$

In example 1 the product obtained by multiplying the denominators (4×5) is 20. Twenty is the lowest multiple of both 4 and 5; therefore 20 will become the denominator of the equivalent fractions. In example 2 it can be seen at once that 18 is a multiple of 6 and that the denominators of the equivalent fractions will be 18.

CHANGING THE FORM OF FRACTIONS

Complex fractions

A complex fraction is another way to indicate division of fractions.

EXAMPLES:

1. $\dfrac{^4/_5}{^8/_9}$ indicates $^4/_5 \div {}^8/_9$
2. $\dfrac{^1/_2}{5}$ indicates $^1/_2 \div 5$
3. $\dfrac{6^2/_3}{3^1/_4}$ indicates $6^2/_3 \div 3^1/_4$

Mixed numbers

To change a mixed number to an improper fraction, multiply the whole number by the denominator, add the numerator to the product, and place the result over the denominator.

EXAMPLES:

1. $3\frac{2}{10} = \dfrac{3 \times 10 + 2}{10}$ or $\dfrac{32}{10}$, an improper fraction
2. $5\frac{1}{6} = \dfrac{5 \times 6 + 1}{6}$ or $\dfrac{31}{6}$
3. $66\frac{2}{3} = \dfrac{66 \times 3 + 2}{3}$ or $\dfrac{200}{3}$

Improper fractions

To change an improper fraction to a mixed number, reduce the fraction by dividing the numerator by the denominator and place the remainder over the denominator.

EXAMPLES:

1. $^{79}/_8 = 79 \div 8$ or $9^7/_8$, a mixed number
2. $^{100}/_3 = 100 \div 3$ or $33^1/_3$
3. $^{47}/_5 = 47 \div 5$ or $9^2/_5$

ADDITION OF FRACTIONS

To add common fractions that have **like denominators,** add the numerators and place over the common denominator

EXAMPLE: $\frac{2}{7} + \frac{4}{7} = \frac{2+4}{7}$ or $\frac{6}{7}$

To add fractions that have **unlike denominators,** change the fractions to equivalent fractions with a common denominator, add the numerators, and place over the common denominator. A mixed number may be changed to an improper fraction before working the problem. Reduce the answer to lowest terms.

EXAMPLES:

1. $^1/_4 + {}^1/_6$ LCM of 4 and 6 is 12

   $\frac{1}{4} = \frac{3}{12}, \frac{1}{6} = \frac{2}{12}; \frac{3+2}{12}$ is $\frac{5}{12}$

2. $2^1/_4 + 4^5/_6$ LCM of 4 and 6 is 12

   $2^1/_4$ and $4^5/_6$ stated as improper fractions are $^9/_4$ and $^{29}/_6$

   $\frac{9}{4} = \frac{27}{12}, \frac{29}{6} = \frac{58}{12}; \frac{27+58}{12}$ is $\frac{85}{12}$ or $7^1/_{12}$

When the mixed number is not changed to an improper fraction, change the unlike fractions to equivalent fractions and add. Then add the product to the whole numbers.

$$\frac{1}{4} = \frac{3}{12}, \frac{5}{6} = \frac{10}{12}; \frac{3+10}{12} \text{ is } \frac{13}{12} \text{ or } 1^1/_{12}$$

$$2 + 4 + 1^1/_{12} = 7^1/_{12}$$

SUBTRACTION OF FRACTIONS

To subtract fractions, change to equivalent fractions if necessary. Subtract the smaller numerator from the larger numerator and place the result over the common multiple.

In subtraction as well as in addition, the same principle applies in changing mixed numbers to improper fractions.

EXAMPLES:

1. $^2/_3 - {}^5/_9$ LCM of 3 and 9 is 9

   $\frac{2}{3} = \frac{6}{9}; \frac{6-5}{9}$ is $\frac{1}{9}$

2. $1\frac{5}{9} - \frac{2}{3}$ LCM of 9 and 3 is 9

$$1\frac{5}{9} = \frac{14}{9},\ \frac{2}{3} = \frac{6}{9},\ \frac{14-6}{9} \text{ is } \frac{8}{9} \quad \text{or} \quad \frac{5}{9} - \frac{2}{3} = \frac{5}{9} - \frac{6}{9}$$

Because the fraction to be subtracted is larger than that from which it is to be subtracted, the whole number is added to the fraction ($1 + \frac{5}{9} = \frac{14}{9}$) and then the subtraction is carried out: $\frac{14}{9} - \frac{6}{9} = \frac{8}{9}$.

MULTIPLICATION OF FRACTIONS

To multiply fractions, multiply the terms of the numerators and then the terms of the denominators. Place the product of the numerators over the product of the denominators. Reduce to lowest terms.

EXAMPLES:

1. $\frac{1}{2} \times \frac{4}{7} = \frac{1 \times 4}{2 \times 7} = \frac{4}{14}$, reduced $= \frac{2}{7}$
2. $2 \times \frac{2}{3} = \frac{2 \times 2}{3} = \frac{4}{3}$, reduced $= 1\frac{1}{3}$

This operation can be shortened by cancelling numbers.

Rule: Factors common to the expressions above and below the line may be divided, or "cancelled out."

EXAMPLE: $\frac{1}{\not{2}} \times \frac{\overset{2}{\not{4}}}{7} = \frac{2}{7}$

To prove, divide the product by the multiplier; the result equals the multiplicand.

$$\frac{2}{7} \div \frac{4}{7} = \frac{\not{2}}{\not{7}} \times \frac{\overset{1}{\not{7}}}{\underset{2}{\not{4}}} = \frac{1}{2}, \text{ the multiplicand}$$

DIVISION OF FRACTIONS

To divide fractions, invert the divisor and multiply.

EXAMPLES:

1. $\frac{6}{9} \div \frac{1}{2} = \frac{6 \times 2}{9 \times 1} = \frac{12}{9}$, reduced $= 1\frac{1}{3}$
2. $8 \div \frac{1}{4} = \frac{8 \times 4}{1 \times 1} = \frac{32}{1}$, reduced $= 32$
3. $\frac{1}{4} \div 8 = \frac{1 \times 1}{4 \times 8} = \frac{1}{32}$
4. $6\frac{1}{2} \div \frac{1}{2} = \frac{13}{\underset{1}{\not{2}}} \times \frac{\overset{1}{\not{2}}}{1} = 13$

To prove, multiply the product by the divisor; the result equals the dividend.

EXAMPLE: Proving problem 3.

$$\frac{1}{\overset{}{\underset{4}{\cancel{32}}}} \times \frac{\overset{1}{\cancel{8}}}{1} = \frac{1}{4}, \text{ the dividend}$$

RATIO

Ratio indicates the relationship of one quantity to another. The quantities must be expressed in the same unit of measure. A ratio is an indicated division or fraction. Therefore the principles that apply to division or to a fraction apply to a ratio.

In changing a fraction to a ratio, the numerator is the first term and the denominator is the second term. The sign of the colon is placed between the two numbers. When changing a ratio to a fraction, the first term in the ratio becomes the numerator and the second term becomes the denominator.

EXAMPLE: $\frac{3}{9}$ expressed as a ratio is 3:9 and is read 3 is to 9.

Both terms of a ratio can be multiplied or divided by the same number without changing the value of the ratio.

EXAMPLE: 3:9 divided by 3 is 1:3; therefore 3:9 equals 1:3.

PROBLEMS

Name ______________________

Date ______________________

FRACTIONS AND RATIO

Change to improper fractions:

1. $3\frac{2}{5}$ =

2. $20\frac{2}{3}$ =

3. $33\frac{1}{3}$ =

4. $3\frac{3}{8}$ =

5. $16\frac{3}{4}$ =

6. $2\frac{2}{3}$ =

Change to mixed numbers:

1. $\frac{26}{3}$ =

2. $\frac{163}{8}$ =

3. $\frac{177}{4}$ =

4. $\frac{13}{2}$ =

5. $\frac{96}{7}$ =

6. $\frac{69}{5}$ =

Add these fractions:

1. $\frac{1}{2} + \frac{1}{3}$ =

2. $\frac{2}{5} + \frac{3}{4} + \frac{5}{12}$ =

3. $\frac{7}{8} + \frac{1}{6} + \frac{1}{2}$ =

4. $\frac{5}{9} + \frac{3}{7} + \frac{1}{3}$ =

Add these fractions—cont'd

5. $4\frac{7}{12} + 9\frac{5}{9} + 1\frac{3}{4} =$

6. $3\frac{1}{3} + \frac{1}{9} =$

Subtract these fractions:

1. $\frac{7}{9} - \frac{2}{3} =$

4. $1\frac{3}{8} - \frac{1}{4} =$

2. $3\frac{5}{8} - \frac{1}{2} =$

5. $\frac{4}{5} - \frac{4}{7} =$

3. $4\frac{3}{8} - 2\frac{1}{16} =$

6. $\frac{1}{100} - \frac{1}{1000} =$

Multiply and reduce answers to lowest terms:

1. $\frac{1}{4} \times \frac{4}{9} =$

3. $2\frac{5}{8} \times 1\frac{3}{5} =$

2. $\frac{1}{1000} \times \frac{1}{10} =$

4. $1\frac{1}{2} \times 2\frac{2}{3} =$

PROBLEMS

Name ______________________

Date ______________________

FRACTIONS AND RATIO—cont'd

Multiply and reduce answers to lowest terms—cont'd

5. $\frac{3}{4} \times \frac{1}{8} \times 2 =$

6. $\frac{1}{5} \times \frac{1}{2} \times \frac{5}{8} =$

Divide and reduce to lowest terms:

1. $\frac{8}{9} \div \frac{2}{3} =$

2. $\frac{1}{150} \div \frac{1}{50} =$

3. $5\frac{1}{5} \div \frac{1}{5} =$

4. $\dfrac{\frac{2}{3}}{\frac{1}{8}} =$

5. $\dfrac{\frac{1}{100}}{\frac{1}{1000}} =$

6. $\dfrac{15}{\frac{1}{2}} =$

Change to ratio in lowest terms:

1. $\frac{1}{8} =$

2. $\dfrac{\frac{1}{4}}{100} =$

3. $\frac{100}{1000} =$

4. $\frac{120}{147} =$

Change ratio to lowest terms—cont'd

5. $\dfrac{33\frac{1}{3}}{66\frac{2}{3}} =$

6. $\dfrac{\frac{2}{3}}{\frac{3}{8}} =$

Change to fractions in lowest terms:

1. 7:49 =

2. 1:100 =

3. 12:40 =

4. 25:200 =

5. 6:252 =

6. 600:6000 =

CHAPTER 3

Decimals

OBJECTIVES

At the completion of this chapter, the student will:

- compute decimal problems
- convert decimals to common fractions and ratios
- convert common fractions to decimals

A decimal fraction is a decimal number indicating a denominator of 10 or power of 10. The numerator is expressed and the denominator is indicated by a period, called a decimal point.

A decimal number having a value less than 1 is a pure decimal fraction.

EXAMPLE: 0.25.

A decimal number having a value more than 1 is a mixed decimal number.

EXAMPLE: 1.25.

Hundred millions	Ten millions	Millions	Hundred thousands	Ten thousands	Thousands	Hundreds	Tens	Units	• - - - - Decimal point	Tenths	Hundredths	Thousandths	Ten thousandths	Hundred thousandths	Millionths	Ten millionths	Hundred millionths
	8	7	6	5	4	3	2	1		1	2	3	4	5	6	7	8

Whole numbers (left of the decimal point) — Decimal fractions (right of the decimal point)

Observe the scale. All whole numbers are to the left of the decimal point, and the place values are ones, tens, hundreds, and so on; all fractions are to the right of the decimal point, and their place values are tenths, hundredths, thousandths, and so on.

To read the decimal numbers read (1) the whole number, (2) the decimal point as "and" or "point," and (3) the decimal fraction.

EXAMPLE:

0.6, read as six-tenths

0.75, read as seventy-five hundredths

125.037, read as one hundred twenty-five and thirty-seven thousandths

In the examples in which the decimal number is less than one, a zero has been placed to the left of the decimal point. This is done in pure decimal fractions to prevent errors resulting from a poorly made decimal point.

Read the following numbers:

1. 978.55
2. 9.1
3. 2.0005
4. 42.001
5. 42.0001
6. 0.037
7. 0.21
8. 0.8756
9. 0.9
10. 0.15341

Underscore the decimal fraction that has the least value:

1. 0.42, 0.042, 0.84
2. 0.01, 0.001, 0.0001
3. 0.3, 0.5, 0.9
4. 0.0007, 0.0075, 0.007
5. 0.7, 0.14, 0.0022
6. 0.3, 0.33, 0.333
7. 0.75, 0.25, 0.85
8. 0.4, 0.6, 0.12
9. 0.25, 0.65, 0.75
10. 0.15, 0.115, 0.1

The same arithmetic processes are carried out with decimal numbers as with other fractions.

ADDITION OF DECIMALS

Write the numbers to be added so that the numerals of the same value are in the same column. Place the decimal point in the sum to the left of the tenths decimal place.

EXAMPLE: 167.094 + 45.51 + 48.1392 =

$$\begin{array}{r} 167.094 \\ 45.51 \\ 48.1392 \\ \hline 260.7432 \end{array}$$

The answer is read as follows: Two hundred sixty and seven thousand four hundred thirty-two ten-thousandths.

SUBTRACTION OF DECIMALS

Write the numbers to be subtracted so that the numerals of the same value are in the same column. Proceed as in subtraction of whole numbers and place the decimal point in the answer to the left of the tenths decimal place.

EXAMPLE: 7453.86 − 391.624 =

$$\begin{array}{r} 7453.86 \\ -\ 391.624 \\ \hline 7062.236 \end{array}$$

The answer is read as follows: Seven thousand sixty-two and two hundred thirty-six thousandths.

MULTIPLICATION OF DECIMALS

Multiply as in whole numbers and point off as many decimal places in the product (beginning from the right) as the sum of the decimal places in the factors (the multiplicand and multiplier).

EXAMPLE: Multiply 562.01 by 7.108

```
     562.01
  ×   7.108
  ---------
     449608
    562010
  393407
  ---------
 3994.76708
```

The answer is read: Three thousand, nine hundred ninety-four and seventy-six thousand, seven hundred eight hundred-thousandths.

To prove, divide the product by the multiplier; the result will equal the multiplicand.

Multiplying a whole number or decimal fraction by 0.1 moves the decimal point one place to the **left;** by 0.01, two places to the left; by 0.001, three places to the left, and so on. If necessary, zeros are prefixed.

EXAMPLE: 42.3 × .1 = 4.23; 42.3 × 0.01 = 0.423; 42.3 × 0.001 = 0.0423.

Multiplying by 10, 100, 1000, and so on moves the decimal point, 1, 2, 3, and so on places to the **right,** respectively.

EXAMPLE: 42.3 × 10 = 423; 42.3 × 100 = 4230; 42.3 × 1000 = 42,300.

DIVISION OF DECIMALS

In dividing by a decimal number, place a caret (‸) as many places to the right of the decimal point in both the divisor and dividend as there are places in the divisor. Place the decimal point in the quotient above the caret in the dividend.

EXAMPLES:

1. Divide 253.680 by 10.5

```
             24.16
10.5‸  ) 253.6‸80
         210
          436
          420
           168
           105
            630
            630
```

2. Divide 50.2990 by 0.125

```
              402.4
0.125‸  ) 50.299‸0
          50 0
             299
             250
              490
              490
```

To prove: The divisor multiplied by the quotient equals the dividend.

If the number of decimal places in the dividend is less than the number in the divisor, add as many zeros to the dividend as necessary.

Dividing by 0.1 moves the decimal point one place to the **right;** by 0.01, two places to the right; by 0.001, three places to the right, and so on. Zeros may be added as necessary.

EXAMPLE: 584.3 ÷ 0.1 = 5843; 584.3 ÷ 0.01 = 58,430; 584.3 ÷ 0.001 = 584,300.

Dividing by 10, 100, 1000, and so on moves the decimal point 1, 2, 3, and so on places to the **left** respectively.

EXAMPLE: 584.3 ÷ 10 = 58.43; 584.3 ÷ 100 = 5.843; 584.3 ÷ 1000 = 0.5843.

CONVERSION OF DECIMALS TO COMMON FRACTIONS AND RATIO

1. To change a decimal fraction to a common fraction, use the number expressed in the decimal fraction as the numerator and the number represented by the decimal place as the denominator.

EXAMPLES: Change 0.8, 0.88, and 0.584 to common fractions.

$0.8 = 8/10 = 4/5$ $\quad$ $0.88 = 88/100 = 22/25$ $\quad$ $0.584 = 584/1000 = 73/125$

2. To change a decimal fraction to a ratio, use the number expressed in the decimal fraction as the first term of the ratio and the number represented by the decimal place as the second term of the ratio; or change decimal fraction to common fraction and change to ratio.

EXAMPLE: $0.5 = 5:10$ or $1:2$ or $0.5 = 5/10 = 1/2$ or $1:2$

Change the decimal in column 1 to common fraction and ratio. Reduce to lowest terms.

	Decimal	Common fraction	Ratio
1.	0.00025		
2.	0.0025		
3.	0.33⅓		
4.	0.05		
5.	0.065		
6.	0.202		
7.	0.025		
8.	0.1045		
9.	0.01		
10.	0.1		
11.	0.001		
12.	0.44		
13.	0.775		
14.	0.92		

CONVERSION OF COMMON FRACTIONS TO DECIMALS

To change a common fraction to a decimal fraction, divide the numerator of the fraction by the denominator of the fraction and express decimally.

EXAMPLE: Change 2/5 to a decimal fraction. $2 \div 5,\quad 5\overline{)2.0}$ = 0.4

PROBLEMS

Name ______________________________

Date ______________________________

DECIMALS

Addition

1. 517.68 + 83.1 + 42.208 =

2. 764.391 + 48.0037 + 90.0095 =

3. 1.66 + 5.101 + 35.907 =

4. 0.1 + 0.135 + 0.025 + 0.125 + 0.65 =

5. 1.0007 + 2357.803 + 2.2 =

6. 15.5 + 0.065 + 0.125 + 30.01 =

7. 1.045 + 0.007 + 4.003 + 5.5 =

8. 26.0275 + 2.002 + 678.4 =

9. 22.27 + 3.03 + 5114 =

10. 0.96 + 0.824 + 0.6 =

Subtraction

1. 2071.3 − 125.25 =

2. 14.825 − 5.224 =

3. 1.5 − 0.75 =

4. 1 − 0.065 =

5. 205 − 9.85 =

8. 56.421 − 8.123 =

6. 98.125 − 10.798 =

9. 0.832 − 0.014 =

7. 3 − 1.175 =

10. 100 − 0.101 =

Multiplication

1. 375.2 × 0.004 =

5. 0.0035 × 7.5 =

2. 363.42 × 0.8 =

6. 14 × 2.04 =

3. 225.5 × 4.001 =

7. 500 × 0.065 =

4. 35.123 × 0.11 =

8. 0.125 × 0.015 =

PROBLEMS

Name ____________________

Date ____________________

DECIMALS—cont'd

9. $745.29 \times 100 =$

10. $0.01 \times 0.001 =$

Division

1. $44.32 \div 0.01 =$

6. $7.623 \div 10.5 =$

2. $18.54 \div 0.5 =$

7. $1.5 \div 0.75 =$

3. $0.34752 \div 0.064 =$

8. $0.376 \div 0.08 =$

4. $0.56 \div 0.002 =$

9. $253.746 \div 1.8 =$

5. $2.5 \div 0.0075 =$

10. $2.272 \div 0.0016 =$

Conversion to decimals

Carry out to fourth decimal place, if necessary.

1. $\frac{5}{8}$ =

2. $\frac{1}{10}$ =

3. $\frac{1}{1000}$ =

4. $\frac{2}{9}$ =

5. $\frac{3}{25}$ =

6. $\frac{3}{7}$ =

7. $\frac{1}{75}$ =

8. $\frac{3}{15}$ =

9. $\frac{1}{500}$ =

10. $\frac{1}{250}$ =

PROBLEMS

Name ______________________

Date ______________________

DECIMALS—cont'd

Conversion of decimals to common fractions and ratio

Reduce to lowest terms:

	Decimal	Common fraction	Ratio
1.	0.105		
2.	0.5		
3.	0.05		
4.	0.33⅓		
5.	0.33		
6.	0.0088		
7.	0.00055		
8.	0.7		
9.	0.464		
10.	0.225		

CHAPTER 4

Percentage and Proportion

OBJECTIVES

At the completion of this chapter, the student will:

- change percent to common fraction, decimal fraction, and ratio
- change common fraction, decimal fraction, and ratio to percent
- determine the given percent of a number
- calculate proportion problems

Percentage

The term **percent** and its corresponding symbol, %, means hundredths. A percent number is a fraction whose numerator is expressed and whose denominator is understood to be 100. The numerical quantity expressed tells how many parts of 100 parts are being considered.

EXAMPLES:

1. $\frac{1}{2}$% means $\frac{1}{2}$ of 1 part of 100 parts is being considered.
2. 5% means 5 parts are being considered.

Percent means hundredths. Hundredths is also expressed by a fraction, a decimal fraction, and a ratio. Therefore a percent number can be changed to a common fraction, decimal fraction, ratio, and vice versa. The form is changed, but the value remains the same.

EXAMPLES:

5% = $\frac{5}{100}$, a fraction

5% = 0.05, a decimal

5% = 5:100, a ratio

CHANGING PERCENT TO COMMON FRACTION, DECIMAL FRACTION, AND RATIO

Percent to common fraction

Remove the % sign and express as hundredths. The numerical quantity will be the numerator and the denominator will be 100. Reduce to lowest terms.

EXAMPLES:

1. $\frac{1}{2}\% = \frac{\frac{1}{2}}{100}$, reduced is $\frac{1}{2} \div \frac{100}{1} = \frac{1}{2} \times \frac{1}{100} = \frac{1}{200}$

2. 5% = 5/100, reduced is 1/20

3. $6\frac{2}{3}\% = \frac{20/3}{100}$, reduced is $\frac{20}{3} \div \frac{100}{1} = \frac{\cancel{20}}{3} \times \frac{1}{\cancel{100}_{5}} = \frac{1}{15}$

Percent to decimal fraction

Percent always has an indicated denominator of 100. If the number (which represents the numerator) is divided by 100, the decimal fraction is quickly obtained. Drop the % sign, count two places to the left, and place the decimal point.

EXAMPLES:

25% = 0.25

1% = 0.01

½% = 0.00½ or 0.005

Alternate method: Remove the % sign and express as a fraction reduced to its lowest terms; dividing the numerator by the denominator gives the decimal fraction.

EXAMPLES:

1. 20% = 20/100, reduced = 1/5; 1 ÷ 5 gives the decimal fraction 0.2
2. 2% = 2/100, reduced = 1/50; 1 ÷ 50 gives the decimal fraction 0.02

In a percent of less than one, such as ½%, and in a mixed percent, such as 6½%, the common fraction does not have a place value.

EXAMPLES:

6½% changed to decimal fraction is 0.06½ or 0.065

½% changed to a decimal fraction is 0.00½% or 0.005

Percent to ratio

The expressed numerator is the first term of the ratio, and the understood denominator (100) is the second term of the ratio. The terms of the ratio should be reduced to lowest terms.

EXAMPLE: 25% = 25:100 or 1:4

CHANGING COMMON FRACTION, DECIMAL FRACTION, AND RATIO TO PERCENT

Common fraction to percent

Multiply the fraction by 100 and add the % sign.

EXAMPLES:

1. ½ changed to % is $\frac{1}{\cancel{2}} \times \overset{50}{\cancel{100}} = 50$; add % sign = 50%

2. 3/200 changed to % is $\frac{3}{\underset{2}{\cancel{200}}} \times \cancel{100} = \frac{3}{2}$ or 1½; add % sign = 1½%

3. $^{30}/_{20}$ changed to % is $\frac{30}{\cancel{20}} \times \overset{5}{\cancel{100}} = 150$; add % sign = 150%

Ratio to percent

Change the ratio to a common fraction and proceed in the same manner as for changing a common fraction to percent.

EXAMPLES:

1. 1:10 = $^1/_{10}$; $\frac{1}{\cancel{10}} \times \overset{10}{\cancel{100}} = 10$; add % sign = 10%
2. 1:500 = $^1/_{500}$; $\frac{1}{\underset{5}{\cancel{500}}} \times \cancel{100} = \frac{1}{5}$; add % sign = $^1/_5$%

Decimal fraction to percent

Use the principle of multiplying by 100. Move the decimal point two places to the right and add the % sign; or change the decimal fraction to a common fraction and proceed the same as for changing common fraction to percent.

EXAMPLES:

1. To change 0.75 to %, move the decimal point two places to right, and add %; the result = 75%
2. To change 0.66⅔ to %, move the decimal point two places to the right, and add %; the result = 66⅔% or 66.6+%.
3. To change 0.0025 to %, move the decimal point two places to the right, and add %; the result = 0.25% or ¼%.

If the percentage does not terminate in a round number, it can be expressed by one of three ways: (1) with the remainder as a common fraction, (2) to the nearest whole percent, or (3) to the nearest tenth of a percent.

EXAMPLES:

⅛ = 12½%

⅛ = 13%

⅛ = 12.5%

FINDING WHAT PERCENT ONE NUMBER IS OF ANOTHER

To find what percent one number is of another number, set up a fraction with the number following the word "of" as the denominator, and the other number the numerator. Divide the numerator by the denominator, multiply by 100, and add the % sign.

EXAMPLES:

1. What % of 50 is 10?

$$\frac{10}{50} = 0.2$$

$0.2 \times 100 = 20$; add % sign = 20%

2. What % of 25 is 35?

$$\frac{35}{25} = 1.40$$

$1.40 \times 100 = 140$; add % sign $= 140\%$

To prove: Change the percent to a decimal fraction or a common fraction. Multiplying by the denominator of the original fraction gives the numerator of the original fraction.

1. $20\% = 0.2;\ \overset{5}{\cancel{50}} \times \frac{2}{\cancel{10}} = 10$

2. $140\% = 1.40;\ \cancel{25} \times \frac{140}{\underset{4}{\cancel{100}}} = 35$

FINDING GIVEN PERCENT OF A NUMBER

To find a given percent of any number, express the percent either as a common fraction or a decimal fraction and multiply by the number.

EXAMPLE: What is 8% of 500?

1. $8\% = 0.08$

$$\begin{array}{r} 500 \\ \times\ 0.08 \\ \hline 40.00 \end{array}$$

2. $8\% = 8/100$

$$\frac{8}{\cancel{100}} \times \overset{5}{\cancel{500}} = 40$$

Proportion

Proportion shows the relationship between two ratios that are equal. The terms of the first ratio are related in the same way as the terms of the second ratio. A proportion may be written in any of the following ways:

1. $8:16 = 1:2$
2. $8:16::1:2$
3. $8/16 = 1/2$

Read as follows: 8 is to 16 equals 1 is to 2, 8 is to 16 as 1 is to 2, or as a fraction, eight-sixteenths equal one-half.

The first and fourth terms of a proportion are called the extremes, and the second and third terms, the means.

Extremes

$8:16::1:2$

Means

In a proportion the product of the means equals the product of the extremes.

If the ratio between two quantities is to be found, the quantities must be expressed in the same unit of measure. The terms of the ratio in the proportion must correspond in value.

x is commonly used to express the unknown terms and for convenience is placed to the left of the equation.

To find the value of an unknown term in a proportion, use the following procedure:

1. Obtain the product of the means and the product of the extremes.
2. Set up the equation.
3. Solve the equation by dividing the terms of the entire equation by the number before the x. This gives the value of x.

EXAMPLE: $3:5::x:10$

$5x$ = product of the means

30 = product of the extremes

$5x = 30$ is the new equation

$5 \,\underline{|\, 5x = 30}$ divide the new equation by the number before the x

$1x = 6$ substituting 6 for x, the proportion reads $3:5::6:10$

Proof: The product of the means = the product of the extremes.

$3 \times 10 = 30$

$5 \times 6 = 30$

Therefore the solution $x = 6$ is correct. If the product of the means does not equal the product of the extremes, an error in setting up the proportion or in mathematics is indicated.

When only a part of the term is unknown, the remaining part can be found in the same manner. In the following example, $x + 1$ is the term and both x and 1 must be multiplied by 10 to get the product of the extremes.

EXAMPLE: $x + 1:12::6:10$

$10 \,\underline{|\, 10x + 10 = 72}$

$1x + 1 = 7.2$

If $x + 1 = 7.2$, $x = 7.2 - 1$, or 6.2

Proof: $7.2:12::6:10$

$7.2 \times 10 = 72$

$12 \times 6 = 72$

Therefore $x + 1 = 7.2$ is correct.

In a proportion expressed in fractions the cross products are equal. The numerator of the first fraction times the denominator of the second fraction equals the denominator of the first fraction times the numerator of the second fraction. The numerator in the first fraction and the denominator of the second fraction correspond to the extremes; the denominator of the first fraction and the numerator of the second fraction correspond to the means.

EXAMPLE: $$\frac{\text{extreme}}{\text{mean}} = \frac{\text{mean}}{\text{extreme}}$$

Therefore we see that the cross products of the fractions are equal.

EXAMPLE: $$\frac{8}{16} = \frac{1}{2}$$

$8 \times 2 = 16$

$16 \times 1 = 16$

If one term in a proportion written as a fraction is missing, it can be found by substituting x, obtaining the cross products, and solving the equation.

EXAMPLE: $\frac{3}{21} = \frac{5}{x}$

$$3x = 105$$

$$3 \underline{\lfloor 3x = 105}$$

$$x = 35$$

$$\therefore \frac{3}{21} = \frac{5}{35}$$

Proof: The cross products will be equal.

$3 \times 35 = 105$

$21 \times 5 = 105$

To find the value of an unknown term in a drug problem, the proportion procedure is used.

EXAMPLE: How much 4% solution can be prepared from 5 ml of a 10% solution?

$0.1:0.04::x:5$

$0.04x =$ product of means

$0.5 =$ product of extremes

$0.04x = 0.5$ is the new equation

$$0.04 \underline{\lfloor .04x = 0.5}$$

$$x = 12.5 \text{ ml}$$

Proof: The product of the means equals the product of the extremes.

$0.4 \times 12.5 = 0.5$

$0.1 \times 5 = 0.5$

PROBLEMS

Name ______________________

Date ______________________

PERCENTAGE AND PROPORTION

Change the percent in column 1 to common fraction, decimal fraction, and ratio.

	Percent	Common fraction	Decimal fraction	Ratio
1.	50			
2.	$66\frac{2}{3}$			
3.	$33\frac{1}{3}$			
4.	$2\frac{1}{2}$			
5.	$5\frac{1}{4}$			
6.	11			
7	48			
8.	23			
9.	75			
10.	0.75			
11.	100			
12.	1			
13.	0.1			
14.	10			
15.	2.5			
16.	25			
17.	0.25			
18.	$18\frac{1}{2}$			
19.	95			
20.	$9\frac{2}{3}$			
21.	4			
22.	4.5			
23.	$\frac{1}{8}$			
24.	$\frac{3}{4}$			
25.	$\frac{2}{5}$			

Change to percent:

1. $\frac{3}{10} =$

2. $\frac{3}{4} =$

3. $2\frac{1}{8} =$

4. $\frac{1}{1000} =$

Change to percent—cont'd

5. $^1/_{100}$ =

6. 0.001 =

7. 0.01 =

8. 3.5 =

9. 0.577 =

10. 2:8 =

11. 1:100 =

12. 1000:2000 =

13. $^1/_3$:100 =

14. 30:36 =

What percent of:

1. 40 is 2?

2. 100 is 55?

3. 75 is 25?

4. 250 is 30?

5. 90 is 9?

6. 700 is 7?

7. 500 is 1?

8. 64 is 8?

PROBLEMS

Name ______________________

Date ______________________

PERCENTAGE AND PROPORTION—cont'd

What percent of—cont'd

9. 60 is 12?

10. 450 is 90?

11. 2.5 is 0.5?

12. 480 is 0.192?

13. 2500 is 50?

14. 625 is 25?

Find percent:

1. 0.125% of 42 =

2. 0.9% of 1600 =

3. ½% of 450 =

4. ¼% of 72 =

5. 75% of 555 =

6. 2½% of 75 =

Find percent—cont'd

7. 9.5% of 1000 =

11. 85% of 1000 =

8. 7% of 10 =

12. 35% of 6300 =

9. 1% of 100 =

13. 8% of 735 =

10. ¾% of 8.75 =

14. 2% of 1500 =

Find the value of x:

1. $1:x::6:102$

4. $0.75:1::x:500$

2. $\frac{1}{2}:x::1:10$

5. $\frac{1}{5000}:\frac{1}{1000}::x:50$

3. $25:x::75:3000$

6. $50:x - 1::5:200$

PROBLEMS

Name ______________________

Date ______________________

PERCENTAGE AND PROPORTION—cont'd

Find the value of x—cont'd

7. $\frac{0.10}{0.20} = \frac{x}{200}$

14. $\frac{4}{2000} = \frac{1}{x}$

8. $\frac{1}{200} : 1 :: 4 : x$

15. $1.5 : 100 :: x : 1000$

9. $\frac{1}{6} : x :: \frac{2}{3} : \frac{3}{4}$

16. $9 : x :: 40 : 480$

10. $\frac{9}{x} = \frac{5}{300}$

17. $\frac{0.15}{0.25} = \frac{x}{20}$

11. $\frac{1}{50} = \frac{x}{20}$

18. $10 : 60 :: 8 : x$

12. $12 : x - 1 :: 3 : 30$

19. $\frac{4}{5}\,x : 85 :: 6 : 10$

13. $\frac{50\%}{100\%} = \frac{x}{1000}$

20. $\frac{1}{100} : x :: \frac{1}{200} : 1$

Find drug proportion:

1. There are 2 ounces of drug in 32 ounces (1 quart) of solution. How much drug is in 1 pint? What is the percentage strength of the solution?

____

2. If you dilute 16 ounces of 5% solution to a 2% solution, how many ounces of the 2% solution do you have?

____

3. A graduate has 375 ml of solution containing 12 g of drug. How much drug is in 100 ml?

____

4. How many ml of 20% solution are needed to make 1 quart of 15% solution?

____

5. A graduate contains 400 ml of 20% solution. How much 4% solution will this make?

____

6. Dilute 10 ounces of 100% solution to 40 ounces. What is the percentage strength of the new solution?

____

PROBLEMS

Name ______________________

Date ______________________

PERCENTAGE AND PROPORTION—cont'd

Find drug proportion—cont'd

7. A solution contains 50 mg per milliliter. How many milliliters will contain 10 mg?

   ____

8. How many milliliters of a ¼% solution can be prepared by diluting 250 ml of a 3% solution?

   ____

9. A solution contains 0.25 mg per milliliter. How many milliliters will contain 0.1 mg?

   ____

10. A solution containing 5 million units of penicillin per 10 ml has been prepared. How many units of penicillin will 0.25 ml contain?

   ____

Find drug proportion—cont'd

11. How much sodium nitroprusside must be added to 250 ml to produce a final concentration of 200 mg per 1000 ml?

____

12. A vial contains 400 mg/ml of Mefoxin. How many milliliters are needed to prepare a 2000-mg dose?

____

13. How many milliliters of 95% alcohol are needed to prepare 60 ml of 30% alcohol?

____

14. How many grams of 30% zinc oxide ointment are needed to prepare 45 g of 7.5% ointment?

____

15. Sterile water for injection is added to a vial of Claforan to provide a concentration of 300 mg/ml. How many milliliters are needed to prepare a 1500-mg dose?

____

PART 2

SYSTEMS OF MEASUREMENTS

- Apothecaries' System
- Metric System
- System Conversion and Household Equivalents
- Temperature Measurement

CHAPTER 5

Apothecaries' System

OBJECTIVES

At the completion of this chapter, the student will:

- state apothecaries' units of measurement for weights and liquids
- convert to equivalent units within the apothecaries' system of measurement

The nurse is required to know systems of measurement and their approximate equivalents to accurately perform the function of drug administration.

The systems of weights and measures commonly used are the apothecaries' and metric systems. Because both measures are used, the nurse is required to know both systems and their approximate equivalents and must be able to convert from one system to the other. Household measurements may be used in the home when more accurate and precise measures are unavailable.

The apothecaries' system is an old English system that was brought to America by the British colonialists. It has traditionally been the system of weights and measures in the United States and continues to be used in spite of attempts to replace it with the metric system. The apothecaries' system was based on the **grain,** which was considered the weight of a grain of wheat, and the **minim,** which was considered the quantity of water equal to the grain of wheat. Roman numerals are used to express whole numbers, and fractions are used to express numbers less than one, except for the fraction one half, which is expressed by the symbol "ss."

The grain, dram, and ounce are the units of weight used to measure drugs in the apothecaries' system. The minim, fluid dram, fluid ounce, pint, quart, and gallon are used to measure fluid volume.

Apothecaries' table of weight

60 grains (gr)	=	1 dram (ʒ)
8 drams (ʒ)	=	1 ounce (℥)
12 ounces (℥)	=	1 pound (lb)

Apothecaries' table of liquid measure

60 minims (♏)	=	1 fluid dram (fl ʒ)
8 fluid drams (fl ʒ)	=	1 fluid ounce (fl ℥)
16 fluid ounces (fl ℥)	=	1 pint (pt or O)
32 fluid ounces (fl ℥)	=	1 quart (qt) or 2 pints (pt)
4 quarts (qt)	=	1 gallon (gal)

PROBLEMS

Name ____________________

Date ____________________

APOTHECARIES' SYSTEM

Change to equivalents within the system:

1. ♏ 15 = fl ʒ ________
2. ♏ 60 = fl ʒ ________
3. ♏ 240 = fl ℥ ________
4. gr 30 = ʒ ________
5. gr 960 = ℥ ________
6. gr 15 = ʒ ________
7. fl ʒ 8 = fl ℥ ________
8. fl ʒ ½ = ♏ ________
9. fl ʒ 16 = fl ℥ ________ = ♏ ________
10. fl ℥ ½ = fl ʒ ________ = ♏ ________
11. fl ℥ 32 = qt ________ = fl ʒ ________ = ♏ ________
12. fl ℥ ¾ = fl ʒ ________ = ♏ ________
13. ♏ 480 = fl ʒ ________ = fl ℥ ________
14. ♏ 120 = fl ʒ ________ = fl ℥ ________
15. qt 3 = pt ________ = gal ________
16. gal ½ = pt ________ = qts ________
17. pt 1 = fl ʒ ________ = fl ℥ ________

Change to equivalents within the system—cont'd

18. pt 3 = fl ℥ ________ = qt ________ = gal ________

19. ℥ 16 = lb ________

20. ℥ 2.5 = ʒ ________

21. ℥ 12 = lb ________

22. gr 240 = ʒ ________ = ℥ ________

23. gr 480 = ʒ ________ = ℥ ________

24. gr 180 = ʒ ________ = ℥ ________

25. gr 120 = ʒ ________ = ℥ ________

CHAPTER 6

Metric System

OBJECTIVES

At the completion of this chapter, the student will:

- state the metric units of measurement for liquids, weights, and length
- convert to equivalent units within the metric system

The metric system was developed in France and is currently used by 90% of the world's population, making it the dominant system of measurement. England, the country from which the United States inherited the apothecaries' system, is currently changing to the metric system. Canada, under the direction of the Metric Commission of Canada, is working toward metrication through a four-phase program of investigation, planning, scheduling, and implementation. When England and Canada complete the conversion, all of the industrial nations will be using the metric system, except the United States.

In the United States, the Metric Conversion Act of 1975 provides coordination and guidance in a voluntary conversion to the International Metric System. This law established a United States Metric Board that has three functions: (1) to carry out a program of planning and coordination to metric conversion at all levels of society, (2) to prepare and implement a comprehensive program of planning and coordinating metric conversion, and (3) to conduct research and make recommendations to Congress and the President. Thus the United States has joined the worldwide trend toward a comparatively new system called the modernized metric system of measurement.

The French Academy of Sciences appointed a committee in 1799 to select the unit of length known as the meter. This is one ten-millionth of the distance from the equator to the North Pole measured along the meridian that passes through Paris, France. A platinum bar, representative of this exact length, was then placed in the French Archives.

One tenth of the meter, which is called the decimeter (dm), was cubed to obtain a unit of weight. The weight of one cubic decimeter of distilled water at the temperature of its greatest density (4° C) was selected as the unit of weight known as the kilogram (kg). A weight of platinum equivalent to the above was placed in the French Archives. The gram (g) is one one-thousandth of the standard kilogram.

The International Bureau of Weights and Measures was established in 1875 in Paris by the International Metric Convention. The original platinum bars were reevaluated, and new bars made of platinum iridium were completed in 1888. International standard meter bars and international standard kilogram weights were then prepared and distributed to participating countries.

In the United States the national standard meter and the national standard kilogram are kept in the United States Bureau of Weights and Measures in Washington, D.C.

The value of the metric system lies in its simplicity, accuracy, and flexibility. The prefixes are the same throughout for linear, weight, and capacity tables. Thus the student needs to know only the unit of length, capacity, or weight and then add the prefixes. Use of the decimal system makes the system precise and decreases the possibility of error that is encountered with fractions.

The units of the metric system are based on the decimal system. Prefixes designate the multiple or submultiple of 10 being used.

Micro	= 0.000001	or	one one-millionth
Milli	= 0.001	or	one one-thousandth
Centi	= 0.01	or	one one-hundredth
Deci	= 0.1	or	one-tenth
Deka	= 10 ×	or	10 times as much
Hecto	= 100 ×	or	100 times as much
Kilo	= 1000 ×	or	1000 times as much

The liter is the unit of measurement for liquid volume in the metric system. The gram is the unit of measure of weight in the metric system. The meter is the unit of measure of length in the metric system. Prefixes of the liter, gram, and meter indicate the number of multiples or submultiples being used.

Liquid measures

1 liter (l) = 1000 milliliters (ml)
1000 liters (l) = 1 kiloliter (kl)

Weight measures

1 gram (g) = 1,000,000 micrograms (μg)
1 gram (g) = 1000 milligrams (mg)
1000 grams (g) = 1 kilogram (kg)

Length measures

1 meter (m) = 1000 millimeters (mm)
1000 meters (m) = 1 kilometer (km)

The most commonly used prefixes and the multiplication factors they indicate are summarized as follows:

Weight (gram)		**Volume (liter)**	
1 microgram	= 0.000001 gram	1 milliliter	= 0.001 liter
1 milligram	= 0.001 gram	1 centiliter	= 0.01 liter
1 centigram	= 0.01 gram	1 deciliter	= 0.1 liter
1 decigram	= 0.1 gram	1 liter	= 1 liter
1 gram	= 1 gram	1 dekaliter	= 10 liters
1 dekagram	= 10 grams	1 hectoliter	= 100 liters
1 hectogram	= 100 grams		
1 kilogram	= 1000 grams		

Length (meter)	
1 millimeter	= 0.001 meter
1 centimeter	= 0.01 meter
1 decimeter	= 0.1 meter
1 meter	= 1 meter
1 dekameter	= 10 meters
1 hectometer	= 100 meters
1 kilometer	= 1000 meters

In the administration of drugs, only a few of the metric measures are used. It is essential that the student learn the most frequently used measures and their abbreviations.

Milli means 0.001 ($^1/_{1000}$) of 1 unit. If the unit referred to is the **liter,** a **milliliter** means 0.001 of the liter.

EXAMPLES:

10 ml means 10 × 0.001, or 0.01 of the liter

250 ml means 250 × 0.001, or 0.25 liters

When the unit is the **gram,** the term **milligram** means 0.001 of the gram.

EXAMPLES:

10 mg means 10 × 0.001, or 0.01 of the gram

476 mg means 476 × 0.001, or 0.476 of the gram

1000 mg means 1000 × 0.001, or 1 gram

PROBLEMS

Name ______________________

Date ______________________

METRIC SYSTEM

Change to equivalents within the system:

1. 1000 μg = ______________ mg
2. 150 μg = ______________ mg
3. 800 μg = ______________ mg
4. 0.1 mg = ______________ μg
5. 0.5 mg = ______________ μg
6. 30 mg = ______________ g
7. 4 mg = ______________ g
8. 100 mg = ______________ g
9. 10 mg = ______________ g
10. 1 mg = ______________ g
11. 850 mg = ______________ g
12. 1500 mg = ______________ g
13. 0.006 g = ______________ mg
14. 0.065 g = ______________ mg
15. 1 g = ______________ mg
16. 0.1 g = ______________ mg
17. 15 g = ______________ mg
18. 5 g = ______________ mg
19. 0.5 g = ______________ mg
20. 0.25 g = ______________ mg
21. 1000 g = ______________ kg
22. 100 g = ______________ kg
23. 1500 g = ______________ kg
24. 0.5 kg = ______________ g
25. 0.05 kg = ______________ g
26. 8 kg = ______________ g
27. 500 ml = ______________ l
28. 900 ml = ______________ l
29. 0.1 l = ______________ ml
30. 1.1 l = ______________ ml
31. 1 l = ______________ ml
32. 7 l = ______________ ml
33. 0.7 l = ______________ ml
34. 250 ml = ______________ l
35. 675 ml = ______________ l
36. 5000 ml = ______________ l

Measure your height and record in centimeters.

____

Record in milliliters the amount of fluid you drank in the past 24 hours.

____

CHAPTER 7

System Conversion and Household Equivalents

OBJECTIVES

At the completion of this chapter, the student will:

- state the common apothecaries' and metric equivalents
- convert unit of measurement in apothecaries' to metric system
- convert unit of measurement in metric to apothecaries' system
- state common household measures with approximate apothecaries' and metric equivalents

The apothecaries' and metric systems of weights and measures are both used in expressing the dosage of drugs and the strength of solutions. The drug or solution on hand may not be in the same system of measure as that written on the prescription or drug order. Thus it becomes necessary to know the equivalent quantities in the two systems. Exact equivalents are seldom used by the nurse in preparing solutions or dosage of drugs since they are not practical.

EXAMPLES OF EXACT EQUIVALENTS:

1 grain = 0.0648 gram
1 gram = 15.432 grains
1 milliliter = 16.23 minims

To facilitate computing and measuring the amount of drug to be used, exact equivalents are rounded off, resulting in approximate equivalents. This makes it possible to convert quickly from one system to another. The variation between the exact equivalents and the approximate equivalents is slight and is considered within the margin of safety for drugs by the United States Pharmacopeia–National Formulary.

APPROXIMATE EQUIVALENTS

Learn the following common equivalents, since they are frequently used in the problems in which conversion is necessary.

Apothecaries' system		Metric system
15 or 16 minims (♏)	is equivalent to	1 milliliter (ml)
1 fluid dram (fl ʒ)	is equivalent to	4 milliliters
1 fluid ounce (fl ℥)	is equivalent to	30 milliliters
1 pint (O)	is equivalent to	500 milliliters
1 quart (qt)	is equivalent to	1000 milliliters
1/60 grain	is equivalent to	1 milligram
1 grain (gr)	is equivalent to	0.065 gram
1 grain	is equivalent to	60 milligrams (mg)
1 grain	is equivalent to	60,000 micrograms (μg)
15 or 16 grains (gr)	is equivalent to	1 gram
1 dram (ʒ)	is equivalent to	4 grams (g)
1 ounce (℥)	is equivalent to	30 grams
2.2 or 2.3 pounds (lb)	is equivalent to	1 kilogram (kg)

Fifteen (15) grains and 15 ♏ are the most commonly used equivalents.

Sixteen (16) grains and 16 ♏ are sometimes used. *Example:* when a 32 ♏ scale hypodermic syringe is used.

Remember that all measures must be in the same system and all units must be the same size in a given problem. *Example:* Milliliters must be changed to minims if problem is worked in the apothecaries' system. Therefore it is necessary to know how to convert from one system to another as well as from one unit within a system to another unit within the same system.

Grams are larger than grains so the result of converting grams to grains will be a larger number; the result of converting grains to grams will be a smaller number.

1 g equivalent to 15 gr
1 gr equivalent to 0.065 g

To change grains to grams divide by 15 or multiply by 0.065.

To change grams to grains multiply by 15 or divide by 0.065.

EXAMPLES:

1. Change 60 gr to grams
   $60 \div 15 = 4$ g
   or
   $60 \times 0.065 = 3.9$ g or approximately 4 g
2. Change 3 g to grains
   $3 \times 15 = 45$ gr
   or
   $3 \div 0.065 = 46.1$ gr or approximately 45 gr

Table of metric doses with approximate apothecary equivalents

Metric	Approximate apothecary equivalents	Metric	Approximate apothecary equivalents
	LIQUID MEASURE		
1000 ml	1 quart	3 ml	45 minims
750 ml	$1\frac{1}{2}$ pints	2 ml	30 minims
500 ml	1 pint	1 ml	15 minims
250 ml	8 fluid ounces	0.75 ml	12 minims
200 ml	7 fluid ounces	0.6 ml	10 minims
100 ml	$3\frac{1}{2}$ fluid ounces	0.5 ml	8 minims
50 ml	$1\frac{3}{4}$ fluid ounces	0.3 ml	5 minims
30 ml	1 fluid ounce	0.25 ml	4 minims
15 ml	4 fluid drams	0.2 ml	3 minims
10 ml	$2\frac{1}{2}$ fluid drams	0.1 ml	$1\frac{1}{2}$ minims
8 ml	2 fluid drams	0.06 ml	1 minim
5 ml	$1\frac{1}{4}$ fluid drams	0.05 ml	$\frac{3}{4}$ minim
4 ml	1 fluid dram	0.03 ml	$\frac{1}{2}$ minim
	WEIGHT		
30 g	1 ounce	30 mg	$\frac{1}{2}$ grain
15 g	4 drams	25 mg	$\frac{3}{8}$ grain
10 g	$2\frac{1}{2}$ drams	20 mg	$\frac{1}{3}$ grain
7.5 g	2 drams	15 mg	$\frac{1}{4}$ grain
6 g	90 grains	12 mg	$\frac{1}{5}$ grain
5 g	75 grains	10 mg	$\frac{1}{6}$ grain
4 g	60 grains (1 dram)	8 mg	$\frac{1}{8}$ grain
3 g	45 grains	6 mg	$\frac{1}{10}$ grain
2 g	30 grains ($\frac{1}{2}$ dram)	5 mg	$\frac{1}{12}$ grain
1.5 g	22 grains	4 mg	$\frac{1}{15}$ grain
1 g	15 grains	3 mg	$\frac{1}{20}$ grain
0.75 g	12 grains	2 mg	$\frac{1}{30}$ grain
0.6 g	10 grains	1.5 mg	$\frac{1}{40}$ grain
0.5 g	$7\frac{1}{2}$ grains	1.2 mg	$\frac{1}{50}$ grain
0.4 g	6 grains	1 mg	$\frac{1}{60}$ grain
0.3 g	5 grains	0.8 mg	$\frac{1}{80}$ grain
0.25 g	4 grains	0.6 mg	$\frac{1}{100}$ grain
0.2 g	3 grains	0.5 mg	$\frac{1}{120}$ grain
0.15 g	$2\frac{1}{2}$ grains	0.4 mg	$\frac{1}{150}$ grain
0.12 g	2 grains	0.3 mg	$\frac{1}{200}$ grain
0.1 g	$1\frac{1}{2}$ grains	0.25 mg	$\frac{1}{250}$ grain
75 mg	$1\frac{1}{4}$ grains	0.2 mg	$\frac{1}{300}$ grain
60 mg	1 grain	0.15 mg	$\frac{1}{400}$ grain
50 mg	$\frac{3}{4}$ grain	0.12 mg	$\frac{1}{500}$ grain
40 mg	$\frac{2}{3}$ grain	0.1 mg	$\frac{1}{600}$ grain

1000 μg = 1.0 mg = gr $\frac{1}{60}$	250 μg = 0.25 mg = gr $\frac{1}{250}$
800 μg = 0.8 mg = gr $\frac{1}{80}$	200 μg = 0.2 mg = gr $\frac{1}{300}$
600 μg = 0.6 mg = gr $\frac{1}{100}$	150 μg = 0.15 mg = gr $\frac{1}{400}$
500 μg = 0.5 mg = gr $\frac{1}{120}$	120 μg = 0.12 mg = gr $\frac{1}{500}$
400 μg = 0.4 mg = gr $\frac{1}{150}$	100 μg = 0.1 mg = gr $\frac{1}{600}$
300 μg = 0.3 mg = gr $\frac{1}{200}$	

Reprinted with permission from the United States Pharmacopeia XX–National Formulary XV, 1980. Note: A milliliter is the approximate equivalent of a cubic centimeter.

HOUSEHOLD MEASURES

Household equivalent measures have been established to meet the needs of persons at home where hospital measuring equipment is generally not available. Medicine droppers, spoons, cups, glasses, and so on may vary in size but are considered relatively safe for measuring some medicines, making solutions for external use, and measuring fluid intake and output in the home. When precise measurement is necessary in the home, the pharmacist should be consulted for proper equipment.

Table of household measures with approximate apothecary and metric equivalents

Household measures	Apothecaries' system	Metric system
1 teaspoonful	60 drops (gtts)	4 or 5 ml
1 teaspoonful	1 fluid dram	4 or 5 ml
1 tablespoonful	4 fluid drams	15 or 16 ml
2 tablespoonfuls	1 fluid ounce	30 ml
1 teacupful	6 fluid ounces	180 ml
1 tumblerful	8 fluid ounces	240 ml

PROBLEMS

Name ______________________

Date ______________________

SYSTEM CONVERSION AND HOUSEHOLD EQUIVALENTS

Convert to units in the apothecaries' system without referring to your tables:

1. 4 ml = ♏ ________
2. 3 ml = ♏ ________
3. 0.3 ml = ♏ ________
4. 8 ml = ♏ ________
5. 2 ml = ♏ ________
6. 8 ml = fl ʒ ________
7. 12 ml = fl ʒ ________
8. 30 ml = fl ℥ ________
9. 24 ml = fl ʒ ________
10. 500 ml = pt ________
11. 300 ml = fl ℥ ________
12. 180 ml = fl ℥ ________
13. 750 ml = pt ________
14. 2000 ml = qt ________
15. 10 l = gal ________
16. 2.5 l = qt ________
17. 1000 μg = gr ________
18. 100 μg = gr ________
19. 250 μg = gr ________
20. 500 μg = gr ________
21. 120 g = ℥ ________
22. 4 mg = ʒ ________
23. 1000 g = lb ________
24. 2 kg = lb ________
25. 500 g = lb ________
26. 0.5 g = gr ________
27. 0.6 g = gr ________
28. 0.3 g = gr ________
29. 0.03 g = gr ________
30. 30 mg = gr ________
31. 0.06 g = gr ________
32. 60 mg = gr ________
33. 0.1 g = gr ________
34. 100 mg = gr ________
35. 5 mg = gr ________
36. 1 mg = gr ________

Convert to units in the metric system without referring to your tables:

1. ♏ 15 = ________ ml
2. ♏ 240 = ________ ml
3. ♏ 90 = ________ ml
4. ♏ 120 = ________ ml
5. ♏ 25 = ________ ml
6. gr 1 = ________ mg
7. gr 1 = ________ g
8. gr 10 = ________ mg
9. gr 10 = ________ g
10. gr 30 = ________ g
11. gr 75 = ________ g
12. gr 2 = ________ mg
13. gr $1/5$ = ________ mg
14. gr $1/100$ = ________ mg
15. gr 150 = ________ g
16. gr $1/4$ = ________ mg
17. gr $1/200$ = ________ mg
18. gr $1/150$ = ________ mg
19. gr $1/60$ = ________ mg
20. gr 450 = ________ g
21. gr 1500 = ________ g
22. fl ʒ 2 = ________ ml
23. fl ʒ ¼ = ________ ml
24. fl ʒ 10 = ________ ml
25. fl ℥ 1 = ________ ml
26. fl ℥ 8 = ________ ml
27. pt ½ = ________ ml
28. qt 1 = ________ ml
29. gal 1½ = ________ ml
30. ℥ 1 = ________ g
31. ʒ 8 = ________ g
32. ℥ ½ = ________ g
33. ℥ 12 = ________ g
34. lb 1 = ________ g
35. ℥ 10 = ________ g
36. ʒ 10 = ________ g

Weigh yourself and record in kilograms. ____________

Change to approximate equivalent in household measure:

1. 1 tsp = ________ T
2. 1 tsp = ________ gtts
3. 1 T = ________ fl ℥
4. ½ tumbler = ________ fl ℥

PROBLEMS

Name ____________________

Date ____________________

SYSTEM CONVERSION AND HOUSEHOLD EQUIVALENTS—cont'd

Change to approximate equivalent in household measure—cont'd

5. 1 teacup = ________ fl ℥
6. 4 T = ________ fl ℥
7. 1 tsp = ________ fl ʒ
8. 3 teaspoonfuls = ________ T
9. 120 ml = ________ T
10. 1 fl ʒ = ________ tsp
11. 6 ml = ________ tsp
12. 30 gtts = ________ tsp
13. 2 fl ℥ = ________ T
14. 16 fl ℥ = ________ pt
15. 480 ml = ________ glassful
16. 6 fl ℥ = ________ teacupful
17. 2 fl ʒ = ________ teaspoonfuls
18. 1 fl ℥ = ________ T
19. 20 gtts = ________ tsp
20. 180 ml = ________ teacupful

CHAPTER 8

Temperature Measurement

OBJECTIVES

At the completion of this chapter, the student will:

- convert temperature from Fahrenheit to Celsius scale
- convert temperature from Celsius to Fahrenheit scale

Two scales are used in measuring temperature, the Fahrenheit and Celsius (Fig. 1). The Celsius scale was originally called the centigrade scale. The instrument used is the thermometer. The inner tube of the thermometer contains mercury, which expands and rises in the tube as heat increases, thereby indicating the temperature on the scale.

The Fahrenheit scale is used on most clinical thermometers in the United States. Because some clinical thermometers use the Celsius scale, it is necessary to know how to convert from one scale to the other. The use of metric measures is increasing in the medical sciences, and the Celsius scale thermometer will be more commonly used in hospitals and other health care settings.

On the Fahrenheit scale, the boiling point is 212° and the freezing point is 32°—a range of 180°. On the Celsius scale, the boiling point is 100° and the freezing point is 0°—a range of 100°. The relationship between boiling and freezing on the scales is expressed as 100:180 or 5:9 (simplified). One degree on the Fahrenheit scale is five-ninths of one degree on the Celsius scale.

A relationship exists between freezing points on the Fahrenheit and Celsius scales. Freezing on the Celsius scale is at 0°; freezing on Fahrenheit is at 32°. Therefore the relationship is expressed as Celsius is to Fahrenheit – 32:

$$C:F - 32$$

From these factors a proportion can be set up to be used as the formula by which temperature can be converted from one scale to another.

$$C:F - 32::5:9$$

Notice in the formula that only a part of a term is missing. The student can refer to p. 34 to review the procedure for finding the term in a proportion when only a part of a term is unknown.

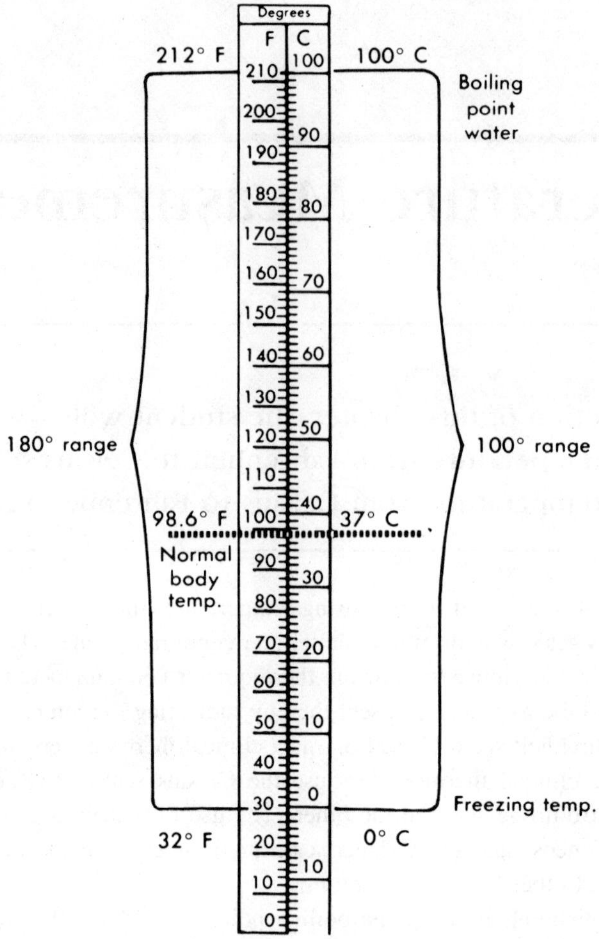

Fig. 1. Scale comparing Fahrenheit and Celsius temperature range.

Substitute the known temperature in a problem and solve for the unknown temperature.

EXAMPLE: Convert 98.6° F to C.

98.6° F is the known temperature, C is the unknown temperature; therefore the problem will read

$$C:98.6 - 32::5:9$$
$$9C = 333$$
$$C = 37 \qquad \therefore 98.6° F = 37° C$$

To prove: Convert 37° C to F.

The problem will read

$$37:F - 32::5:9$$
$$5F - 160 = 333$$
$$5F = 333 + 160, \text{ or } 493$$
$$F = 98.6 \qquad \therefore 37°C = 98.6°F$$

The student may wish to select another method of converting Fahrenheit to Celsius and Celsius to Fahrenheit. There are 100° C and 180° F between ice point and steam point; therefore 100° C = 180° F. Dividing 180 by 100 we find that 1° C = $^9/_5$° F, and 1° F = $^5/_9$° C. Noting that 0° C and 32° F are the same temperature, to convert a temperature in Celsius to Fahrenheit, multiply the Celsius temperature by $^9/_5$ and add 32°:

$$F = {}^9/_5C + 32$$

To convert Fahrenheit to Celsius, multiply $^5/_9$ by the Fahrenheit temperature minus 32.

$$C = {}^5/_9(F - 32)$$

Following are two examples illustrating the use of these formulas:
40° C is an elevated body temperature. Convert to Fahrenheit.

$$F = {}^9/_5C + 32$$
$$F = {}^9/_5 \times 40 + 32$$
$$F = 72 + 32$$
$$F = 104$$

77° F is a comfortable room temperature for ill patients. Convert to Celsius.

$$C = {}^5/_9(F - 32)$$
$$C = {}^5/_9(77 - 32)$$
$$C = {}^5/_9 \times 45$$
$$C = 25$$

PROBLEMS

Name ______________________________

Date ______________________________

TEMPERATURE MEASUREMENT

Convert from one temperature scale to the other:

1. 50° C to F =

2. 113° F to C =

3. 38° C to F =

4. 212° F to C =

5. 0° C to F =

6. 101° F to C =

7. 68° F to C =

8. 60° C to F =

9. 15° C to F =

10. 185° F to C =

Convert from one temperature scale to the other—cont'd

11. The wall thermometer registers the temperature of the room at 72° F. Change to Celsius.

____

12. The physician wishes the temperature of the room to be 68° F. What is this temperature on the Celsius thermometer?

____

13. The normal body temperature is 98.6° F by mouth, one degree higher rectally. What would these temperatures be on the Celsius scale?

a. _______________; b. _______________

14. A patient's temperature is 104° F. What is it when expressed on the Celsius scale?

____

15. A patient's temperature is 40° C. What is it on the Fahrenheit thermometer?

____

PROBLEMS

Name ______________________

Date ______________________

TEMPERATURE MEASUREMENT—cont'd

16. The temperature of the refrigerator is 5° C. Convert to Fahrenheit.

____

17. The temperature of a hot-water bottle is 120° F. What is it in Celsius?

____

18. A tepid bath is 30° C. What is it in Fahrenheit?

____

19. A drug should be stored at 40° to 60° F. What is the range in Celsius?

____

20. A drug should be stored at 2° to 8° C. What is the range in Fahrenheit?

____

PART 3

CALCULATION OF DOSAGE

- Introduction to Dosage
- External Dosage
- Oral Dosage
- Parenteral Dosage
- Pediatric Dosage

CHAPTER 9

Introduction to Dosage

OBJECTIVES

At the completion of this chapter, the student will:

- state terms used to modify the quantity of the dose of a drug
- list common dosage forms
- identify factors that influence the determination of drug dosage
- define abbreviations when interpreting drug orders

Dosage is the determination and regulation of doses. The study of dosage is **posology.**

A dose is the quantity to be administered at one time. Several terms are used to modify this quantity.

Minimum dose small dose that will produce a therapeutic effect
Maximal dose largest dose that can be safely administered
Loading dose quantity to rapidly achieve desired plasma level
Daily dose quantity to be administered in a 24-hour period
Average dose quantity that will usually produce the desired therapeutic effect
Maintenance dose quantity that will maintain the desired therapeutic effect
Toxic dose dose that produces poisonous effects
Lethal dose dose that produces death

The nurse must know correct dosage to administer drugs effectively, recognize errors, and observe therapeutic effects. A possible error in dosage in an order should be referred to the physician for verification or correction.

The pharmacist dispenses drugs in the dosage and dosage form ordered by physicians for patients. A supply of medication may be dispensed that will be adequate for several days. The nurse is responsible for the preparation of each dose at the time of administration. Another dispensing system is called **unit dose.** Each dose of drug is prepared in unit of use form, in the prescribed dose, packaged, labeled, and ready to use. It is delivered to the nursing station by the pharmacy department. The nurse need not prepare the medication in any manner except to open the individual packet dose and administer.

DRUG STANDARDIZATION AND LEGISLATION

To ensure accurate dosage and specific therapeutic effect, drugs must be of uniform strength, have a standard of purity, and be free from harmful substances. National and international drug laws have been established to ensure drug standardization and to protect the consumer against the indiscriminate use of certain drugs and against manufacturers who make excessive or false claims for their products. Control of these factors is established by federal and state laws in the United States. Other countries have similar types of legislation to protect drug consumers. See Appendix A for additional reading and exercises.

FACTORS INFLUENCING DRUG DOSAGE

In determining proper drug dosage, many factors affecting dosage are recognized, including those discussed in the following paragraphs.

Age

Children and older persons are very sensitive to the effects of many drugs and require carefully calibrated smaller doses. This population is vulnerable to drug effects because of lowered body metabolism, decreased body mass, and decreased ability to excrete the drugs. In addition, the hazard of drug interactions, especially in older adults, has an effect on drug dosage.

Sex

Females are considered to be more sensitive to drug action, manifesting more prolonged effects. The need for smaller doses is based on lower body weight and greater proportion of body fat. These differences from males result in slower drug metabolism.

Weight

Usual doses are intended for adult patients with body weights in the average range of 60 to 70 kg (132 to 154 pounds). Doses must be adjusted for persons of very low or relatively high body weight. Obese persons present a problem because many drugs are primarily distributed in the water and lean body mass and not into fat.

Method of administration

The route of administration of a drug has an effect on the rate at which the drug is absorbed. Larger doses are generally used when a drug is administered orally and smaller doses when administered parenterally.

Time of administration

Absorption is affected by the time the drug is administered. For example, the rate of absorption of oral drugs is affected by the absence or presence of food in the stomach.

Pathologic conditions

Pathophysiologic changes in an individual can affect rates of absorption, metabolism, and excretion. Hepatic and renal disease, cardiovascular dysfunction, and presence of infection, pain, or anxiety influence drug dosage.

Absorption and excretion

Drugs that are rapidly excreted are administered at more frequent intervals. If absorption is rapid and excretion is slow, drugs are given at less frequent intervals to prevent accumulation of the drug and possible toxic response.

Repeated dosage

When individuals receive repeated dosage of a drug, various responses may occur. A cumulative effect is a slowly increasing response caused by a rate of dosing that exceeds the rate of excretion. Tolerance, or a decreased response to a drug, may also occur with repeated administration. This response is possibly caused by an alteration in drug metabolism or an adaptation to the drug's action.

Combination of drugs

The effects of one drug may be modified by the presence of another drug. An increased or decreased response may occur with the simultaneous administration of two drugs. An enhanced response, or synergism, may be caused by an additive effect or a potentiating effect. A decreased response, or antagonism, may be caused by competition for receptor site, inactivation of one drug by another, or multiple other causes. Drug interaction information has been compiled as a result of the proliferation of drugs and their combination for patient use.

DOSAGE FORMS

Drugs may be administered in various dosage forms. The dosage form and the method of administration influence the therapeutic effectiveness of the drug. Nurses should be familiar with the preparations that are made by the pharmacist or the company from which they are purchased.

The commonly used dosage forms are described in the following list.

Capsules powdered drugs, oils, or liquids that are within a readily soluble gelatin container.

Tablets powdered drugs that are compressed or molded into small discs.

Elixirs solutions containing alcohol, sugar, and water. They may contain active medicinal ingredients, but more commonly they are used as flavoring agents or solvents.

Syrups aqueous solutions of sugars that may contain medicinal ingredients.

Suppositories mixtures of drugs with a firm base that are molded into shapes suitable for insertion into a body orifice (urethral, vaginal, rectal). The substances melt at body temperature, causing local or systemic effects.

Solutions liquid preparations containing one or more substances that are completely dissolved in solution.

Creams mixtures of one or more drugs in an aqueous base, for external use.

Ointments mixtures of one or more drugs in a fatty base, for external use.

Liniments combinations of drugs with oil, soap, water, or alcohol that are for external application by rubbing on the skin.

Lotions aqueous preparations containing suspended materials that are for external application by gently patting on the skin.

Waters saturated solutions of volatile oils.

Tinctures alcoholic or hydroalcoholic solutions prepared from drugs.

Emulsions dispersions of fat globules in water prepared with the aid of an emulsifying agent.

DRUG ORDERS

Orders for the administration of drugs are written by the physician. In addition to the drug and the dosage, these orders give other information such as when the drug is to be given, how it is to be given, and how many times it is to be given. Orders are written in abbreviated form. To interpret orders for medication, students must thoroughly learn the commonly accepted abbreviations.

Hospitals are required by the Joint Commission on Accreditation of Hospitals to develop a list of pharmaceutical abbreviations and chemical symbols approved by the medical staff for use in the patient medical record. Only abbreviations with a clear meaning should appear on the list.

The table that follows gives a list of commonly used abbreviations. An understanding of these abbreviations is essential for safe medication administration.

In the metric system the amount of drug to be given is written before the metric measure. Arabic and decimal numbers should always be used.

EXAMPLES: 1 g, 0.1 g, 1.8 g, 10 mg, 0.05 mg, 1000 ml, ½ liter

In the apothecaries' system the apothecary measure is usually written before the amount of drug to be given. Arabic and Roman numerals are both used. Decimal numbers are rarely used.

EXAMPLES: gr 5½, gr 3, gr ¾, gr 1/100, ℥ 10, ʒ 4, ♏ 5, ♏ 10

When Roman numerals are used, the I is expressed as i for clarity; the abbreviation ss is often used to express one half (½).

EXAMPLES: gr vss, gr iii, gr xv, gr viiss, ℥ iss, ʒ xii, ♏ xx, ♏ viii

In order for a drug to be administered correctly, the nurse must know the drug, dosage form, route, dose, frequency or rate of administration, and time of administration. If the medication order is improperly written by the physician or is not accurately interpreted by the nurse or pharmacist, medication errors can occur.

Use of abbreviations and obscure terminology has contributed to medication errors, which occur because of unfamiliarity with or the possibility of more than one meaning

Table of abbreviations for prescriptions and orders

Abbreviation	Meaning	Abbreviation	Meaning
aa	of each	o.h. or q.h.	every hour
a.c.	before meals	ol.	oil
ad.	up to	o.m.	every morning
ad lib.	as desired	o.n.	every night
aq.	water	os	mouth
aq. dest.	distilled water	O.S.	in left eye
b.i.d.	twice a day	O.U.	in each eye
c̄	with	oz. or ℥	ounce
caps.	capsules	p.c.	after meals
comp.	compound	per	by
dil.	dilute	pil.	pill
elix.	elixir	p.r.n.	when required
ext.	extract	q. 2 h.	every 2 hours
fld. or fl.	fluid	q. 3 h.	every 3 hours
Ft.	make	q. 4 h.	every 4 hours
g	gram	q.i.d.	four times a day
gr	grain	q.s.	quantity sufficient
gtt.	drop	℞	take
H.	by hypodermic	s	without
h.	hour	s.c.	subcutaneously
h.s.	hour of sleep	Sig.	write on label
I.M.	intramuscularly	sol.	solution
I.V.	intravenously	s.o.s.	once if necessary
M.	mix	sp.	spirits
♏ or m	minim	ss	one half
μg	microgram	stat.	immediately
mg	milligram	t.i.d.	three times a day
mixt.	mixture	tr.	tincture
ml	milliliter	U	unit
O	pint	ung.	ointment
O.D.	in right eye	vin.	wine
o.d. or q.d.	every day		

for the term. Unclear handwriting of the order by physicians adds to the possibility of error in order interpretation by the nurse or pharmacist. The importance of clarifying the order by questioning the physician needs to be stressed to prevent potential errors.

PRESCRIPTIONS

A prescription is an order for medicine written by the physician directing a pharmacist to dispense medication for the patient.

Nurses are sometimes required to read or to copy prescriptions from the chart or order book to be sent to a pharmacy.

A typical prescription consists of the following parts:

1. Superscription—name of patient, address, date, and ℞ (meaning "take thou")
2. Inscription—the ingredients and their amounts
3. Subscription—directions to the pharmacist
4. Signature—the direction to the patient (this is written on the label)
5. The physician's signature and address. If the prescription ingredients contain a drug that is controlled under the Comprehensive Drug Abuse Prevention and Control Act, the physician's registry number must also be on the prescription.

An example of a prescription is shown below. The numbers refer to the parts of the prescription.

1	**Rx** **Mrs. Mary Larson** **4421 N. Oakland Ave.** **St. Louis, MO**
2	**Prednisone 5 mg tabs**
3	**#30**
4	**Sig: 1 bid**
5	**T. Fowler, M.D.** **425 East Monroe** **AF 3932440**

PROBLEMS

Name ____________________

Date ____________________

INTRODUCTION TO DOSAGE

Abbreviation	Meaning	Abbreviation	Meaning
1. aa		31.	every day
2. a.c.		32.	every hour
3.	up to	33. o.m.	
4.	as desired	34. o.n.	
5.	water	35. os	
6. aq. dest.		36.	ounce
7.	twice a day	37. p.c.	
8.	with	38. per	
9. caps.		39. pil.	
10. comp.		40.	when required
11.	dilute	41.	every two hours
12.	elixir	42.	every three hours
13.	extract	43.	every four hours
14. fl.		44.	every six hours
15.	make	45. q.i.d.	
16.	gram	46. q.s.	
17.	grain	47. ℞	
18. gtt.		48.	without
19. H.		49. s.c.	
20. h.		50. Sig.	
21.	hour of sleep	51.	solution
22. I.M.		52. s.o.s.	
23. I.V.		53.	spirits
24. kg		54.	one half
25. M.		55.	immediately
26. mg		56. t.i.d.	
27. ml		57. tr.	
28.	minim	58.	unit
29.	mixture	59. ung.	
30.	pint	60. vin.	

Interpret the following orders:

1. Ampicillin capsules 0.5 g q. 4 h. os.

2. Nitroglycerin gr $^{1}/_{150}$ sublingually stat. and p.r.n.

3. Erythromycin 250 mg tablet t.i.d.

4. Calcium gluconate gr viiss I.M. from an ampule labeled 0.5 g in 2 ml.

5. Synkayvite 10 mg q.d. I.M.

6. Apply lanolin ung. to lips ad lib.

7. Dalmane 15 mg per os, h.s.

8. Aspirin and calcium carbonate gr v aa, stat. and p.r.n.

9. Valium 5 mg per os, stat. and b.i.d.

10. Regular insulin U 10, ½ h., a.c.

PROBLEMS

Name ______________________

Date ______________________

INTRODUCTION TO DOSAGE—cont'd

Interpret the following orders—cont'd

11. Morphine sulfate gr ¼ q. 4 h., H.

12. Apply neomycin solution to wound q. 2 h. for 12 h.

13. Dil. 4 ml procaine solution c̄ sufficient aq. dest. to make 6 ml.

14. Tetracaine ½% gtt. ii in O.S. stat.

15. Elix. terpin hydrate c̄ codeine ʒ i per os, q. 4 h. and p.r.n.

16. Thyroid gr iii per os, q.d.

17. 600,000 U procaine penicillin I.M. b.i.d.

18. Fl. ext. cascara sagrada ʒ ii per os, p.r.n.

19. Elix. Benadryl ʒ iss per os, o.m. and o.n.

Interpret the following orders—cont'd

20. Sodium phenobarbital gr ii s.c., stat.

21. Dil. $\bar{c}$ aq. ♏ xv tr. opium and give per os, a.c., b.i.d.

22. Ferrous sulfate 0.3 g t.i.d. per os $\bar{c}$ meal or p.c.

23. Lanoxin 0.125 mg b.i.d.

24. gtt. i of pilocarpine 1% in O.U., q.d. P.M.

25. Timoptic 0.25% 1 gtt. O.D. q. 12 h.

26. Restoril 15 mg, h.s., may repeat s.o.s.

27. Cold cream and white petrolatum aa 1 oz. M.Ft. ung., apply h.s.

28. Feldene cap. 20 mg, o.m.

29. Isoptocarpine 2% 1 gtt. o.s., q.i.d.

PROBLEMS

Name ______________________

Date ______________________

INTRODUCTION TO DOSAGE—cont'd

Interpret the following orders—cont'd

30. Furosemide 80 mg I.V. q 12 h.

31. Tr camphorated opium 5 ml, 1 to 4 times a day and p.r.n.

32. Dil. 0.5 ml Haldol concentrate $\bar{c}$ ½ oz. vin

33. Serax 15 mg per os, t.i.d.

34. Heparin 5000 U s.c., q.d.

35. Amitriptyline 25 mg 1 h. p.c. and h.s.

CHAPTER 10

External Dosage

OBJECTIVES

At the completion of this chapter, the student will:

- calculate the amount of pure or full strength drug required to make a designated solution
- determine the amount of stock solution required to make a designated solution
- calculate the percentage or ratio strength of solutions

This chapter deals with solutions in relatively large quantities that are used externally in treatments such as medicinal bath packs, irrigations, and stomach lavage. Commonly used solutions can be purchased from pharmaceutical companies or obtained from the pharmacy. However, the nurse should be able to make a large quantity of solution for external use if the need arises and be able to recognize and compute the strength of solutions.

A solution is a clear, homogeneous mixture with no tendency to settle out upon standing. It results from dissolving one or more substances in a liquid. The solution may be a mixture of gases, liquids, or solids in liquid. The nurse focuses attention on liquids in liquids or solids in liquids.

The parts of a solution are the solvent and the solute:

Solvent is the liquid in which the solute is dissolved.

Solute is the substance dissolved.

SOLUBILITY OF DRUGS

Solubility varies with the temperature of the solvent, the pressure, and the composition of the solvent and solute. Soluble substances that dissolve in all proportions are said to be freely soluble. Water is known as the universal solvent because most substances will dissolve in it.

Fatty substances are insoluble in water but are freely soluble in ether, benzene, or gasoline.

Iodine crystals are slightly soluble in water, readily soluble in alcohol. Crystals are less soluble than are powdered substances because less surface is in contact with the solvent. Fewer molecules of the solid are in contact with the molecules of the solvent. Stirring aids the dissolving process.

Temperature affects the solubility of substances, in many instances increasing the action of the solvent, in others producing little or no effect. In a few cases a rise in temperature lessens the solubility of the solute.

Increasing the temperature decreases the solubility of gases in solution. Let a tumblerful of water stand after drawing it from the faucet. In a short time bubbles will appear, showing that the air, which was in solution, is coming out. In preparing solutions that owe their action to gases, this process should be remembered. When pressure is removed from a carbonated solution, such as carbonated magnesium citrate, gas is lost from the solution, and its value is decreased or lost. Such medication should be given as soon as the bottle is opened.

CLASSIFICATION OF SOLUTIONS BASED ON STRENGTH OF SOLUTION

As previously stated, a solution is made up of two parts, the solute and the solvent. The strength of a solution is based on the amount of solute in a given quantity of solution and is expressed either as a percent, fraction, or ratio. In the preparation of solutions and administration of drugs, the nurse is concerned with solutes that are liquid or solids dissolved in liquid (the solvent).

Dilute solutions contain a small amount of the solute in the solution.

Concentrated solutions contain a large amount of the solute in the solution.

Saturated solutions contain all the solute the solution can hold at ordinary temperature and pressure.

Supersaturated solutions hold more of the solute than the solution would hold under ordinary temperature and pressure.

Isotonic solutions are solutions that are of equal concentration. An example is physiologic salt solution, which is isotonic with the blood.

Hypotonic solutions are solutions in which the concentration of solute in one is less than the concentration of solute in the other. Thus a saline solution of 0.6% is hypotonic to the blood, because the salts in the blood are 0.85% (0.9%).

Hypertonic solutions are solutions in which the concentration of solute in one solution is greater than the concentration of solute in the other. A 10% salt solution would be hypertonic to the blood. When 10% salt solution is brought into contact with the red corpuscles of the bloodstream, plasmolysis, shrinking, or crenation will occur.

Colloidal solutions are solutions in which the molecules will pass through filter paper but not through a membrane such as parchment. Glue, white of egg, and acacia are all examples of colloidal solutions. They are opalescent, sticky, translucent substances. Some of the colloidal solutions with which a nurse will come in contact have some or all of these qualities. The mild silver protein preparation 10% Argyrol is an example.

PREPARATION OF SOLUTIONS

Methods of preparing solutions

Weight to weight. A given part by weight of a solute is dissolved in a given number of parts by weight of the solvent. This is the most accurate method of preparation, but it is not commonly used because balances are not available to weigh the drug.

Weight to volume. A given part by weight of a solute is dissolved in a sufficient amount of the solvent to make the required amount of the solution. This method is less exact than weight to weight but is practical for the solutions the nurse is required to prepare.

Volume to volume. A given volume of solute is added to a given volume of solvent.

Types of drug preparations for solutions

The types of drugs used for preparation of solutions are usually those soluble in water. They are either pure drugs or drugs in stock solution.

Pure drugs. Pure drugs are drugs considered to be 100% in strength and are referred to as **full-strength drugs.** They come in the form of crystals, powder, tablets, and liquids. The following list gives examples of pure drugs.

Crystals:
- Boric acid
- Magnesium sulfate
- Carbolic acid or phenol
- Iodine
- Camphor
- Potassium permanganate

Powders:
- Zinc oxide
- Boric acid
- Starch
- Sodium bicarbonate

Tablets:
- Sodium chloride 1 g (gr 15)
- Mercuric chloride 0.5 g (gr 7½)
- Potassium permanganate 0.06, 0.2, or 0.33 g (gr 1, 3, or 5)

Liquids:
- Cresol
- Ethyl alcohol
- Glycerine

Stock solutions. Stock solutions contain the drug diluted in the solvent. These solutions may be 100% or less in strength. The strength of the solution is stated on the label of the bottle. Most solutions are less than 100%. The following are examples of stock solutions:

Alcohol 70%

Tincture iodine 7%

Saturated stock solutions. Saturated stock solutions are so called because they contain all the solute that they can hold. The following are examples of saturated stock solutions:

Saturated solution potassium iodide

Saturated solution magnesium sulfate

PROBLEM ANALYSIS

In solving problems you have known factors and you are asked to find an unknown factor. The inexperienced student needs to study the problem carefully and to make a working plan. The following method of analyzing the problem should be followed until the student becomes skilled in recognizing the factors in the problem.

1. State the factors in the problem:
   a. Strength desired
   b. Strength on hand
   c. Amount of solute
   d. Total amount of solution

   Any one of these factors may be unknown.
2. Check terms in the problem.

All measures and weights in the problem must be expressed either in the apothecaries' system or in the metric system, and strengths must be expressed similarly, percent to percent or ratio to ratio.

If conversions need to be made, the quantity of solution may be a guide in deciding what system of measure to use. Large quantities are usually expressed in milliliters; therefore measures will be in the metric system. Small quantities expressed in minims would require the measures in the problem to be in the apothecaries' system.

Ability to accurately convert to like strengths is important. If necessary, review converting percent to ratio, decimals, and fractions, and vice versa. After you have analyzed the problem, arrange the data, solve the problem, and prove the problem.

Solutions from pure or full-strength drugs

FINDING THE AMOUNT OF DRUG NEEDED TO PREPARE A KNOWN AMOUNT OF SOLUTION OF DESIRED STRENGTH

Problem 1

Prepare 1 liter of 5% boric acid solution.

An analysis of the problem shows the following factors:

$$\begin{aligned} 5\% &= \text{strength desired} \\ 100\% &= \text{strength on hand} \\ x &= \text{amount of solute} \\ 1 \text{ liter} &= \text{total amount of solution} \end{aligned}$$

The boric acid to be used is the crystalline form; therefore the solute will have to be in a unit of weight, either grams or grains; the liter will have to be in the same system of measure as the solute and will be milliliters or minims. When working with a large quantity such as a liter, it is more convenient to use milliliters than minims. The problem will then be solved in the metric system, and the answer will be expressed in grams. The strength of the solution desired and the strength on hand are expressed in percent, so no conversion is necessary. The proportion will be %:% = solute in grams:solution in milliliters, which shows strength: strength:: solute: solution, as well as small: large:: small: large.

Methods for solving the problem

Solving the problem by proportion:

$$5\%:100\% = x \text{ g solute}:1000 \text{ ml solution}$$

Simplify:

$$5\%:100\% = 5:100$$

$$\begin{aligned} 5:100&::x:1000 \\ 100x &= 5000 \\ x &= 50 \end{aligned}$$

$\therefore$ 50 g are needed to make 1 liter.

Proof: When the value of x is substituted in the proportion, the product of the means will equal the product of the extremes if the problem has been worked correctly.

$$\begin{aligned} 5:100&::50:1000 \\ 5000 &= 5000 \end{aligned}$$

Proportions can also be set up as fractions. (Refer to p. 35.) After simplifying 5%: 100%, the problem reads as follows:

$$\begin{aligned} \frac{5}{100} &= \frac{x}{1000} \\ 100x &= 5000 \\ x &= 50 \end{aligned}$$

$\therefore$ 50 g are needed to make 1 liter.

When a proportion is written in fractions, the cross products are equal. The value of x can also be obtained by multiplying the entire first fraction by the denominator of the second fraction.

$$\frac{5}{100} \times 1000 = x$$

$$\frac{5}{\cancel{100}} \times \overset{10}{\cancel{1000}} = 50$$

$\therefore$ 50 g are needed to make 1 liter.

Proof: The product divided by the multiplier equals the multiplicand:

$$50 \div \frac{5}{100} = \overset{10}{\cancel{50}} \times \frac{100}{\cancel{5}} = 1000$$

Analysis of this method shows that the first term or numerator is the strength desired; the second term or denominator is the strength on hand; the third term is the quantity of solution; the fourth term is the amount of solute. Any one of the terms can be unknown and found by substituting x and solving the problem. This is a simple method to use in finding the value of an unknown term. Students should understand and learn this method because it is used in solving drug dosage problems.

$$\frac{\text{strength desired}}{\text{strength on hand}} \times \text{quantity of solution} = \text{amount of solute}$$

Problem 2

Prepare 500 ml of 1:20 strength solution from pure drug. Analyzing the problem shows the factors are as follows:

$$\begin{aligned} 1{:}20 &= \text{strength desired} \\ 100\% &= \text{strength on hand} \\ x &= \text{amount of solute} \\ 500 \text{ ml} &= \text{total amount of solution} \end{aligned}$$

Checking the terms in the problem, note that the strength of the drug desired and the drug on hand are in unlike terms; therefore it is necessary to change the strengths so that both will be either in ratio or percent. It is convenient to change to percent. 1:20 changed to % = 5%. The problem will read as follows:

$$\frac{5\% \text{ strength desired}}{100\% \text{ strength on hand}} \times 500 = x$$

Simplify:

$$\frac{5\%}{100\%} = \frac{5}{100} = \frac{1}{20}$$

$$\frac{1}{\cancel{20}} \times \overset{25}{\cancel{500}} = 25$$

$\therefore$ 25 ml of solute are needed.

To prepare 500 ml of 1:20 strength solution, dilute 25 ml of 100% solution to 500 ml by adding 475 ml of water.

Explanation. When the solute is a liquid, it is part of the total volume of the solution. The amount of solute is measured in a graduate, and water is added to make the total amount of solution required.

When the solute is a solid, it dissolves without replacing volume in the total amount of solution. Therefore the solute is dissolved in the total amount of solution.

Proof: The product divided by the multiplier equals the multiplicand.

$$25 \div \frac{1}{20} = \overset{5}{\cancel{25}} \times \frac{100}{\cancel{5}} = 500$$

Problem 3

Prepare 1000 ml of 1 : 1000 solution from tablets of gr $7\frac{1}{2}$. How many tablets will be needed?

Analyzing the problem shows the factors are as follows:

$$\begin{aligned} 1:1000 &= \text{strength desired} \\ 100\% &= \text{strength on hand} \\ x &= \text{amount of solute} \\ 1000 \text{ ml} &= \text{total amount of solution} \end{aligned}$$

In this problem there are two factors to find—the amount of solute and the number of tablets. First find the amount of solute and then find the number of tablets.

The strength desired and the strength on hand are expressed in unlike terms. A strength on hand of 100% can be expressed as a ratio of 1 : 1, or 1 : 1000 can be expressed in percentage as 0.1%. The drug is in tablet form; therefore the answer will be expressed in a measure of weight. Since the total solution is in milliliters, the problem will be worked in the metric system.

Solve the problem by using (1) the percent conversion and (2) the ratio conversion as follows:

1. $\dfrac{0.1\%}{100\%} \times 1000 = x$

$$\frac{0.1}{\cancel{100}} \times \overset{10}{\cancel{1000}} = x$$

$$x = 1$$

2. $\dfrac{1:1000}{1:1} \times 1000 = x$

$$\frac{1}{\cancel{1000}} \times \overset{1}{\cancel{1000}} = x$$

$$x = 1$$

$\therefore$ 1 g needed

Proof:

1. $1 \div {}^{0.1}/_{100} = 1 \times \dfrac{100}{0.1} = 1000$

2. $1 \div {}^{1}/_{1000} = 1 \times \dfrac{1000}{1} = 1000$

The solute is expressed in gr $7\frac{1}{2}$ (0.5 g) tablets. To find the number of tablets needed, divide the number of grams in the solute by the number of grams in a tablet.

$$1 \text{ g} \div 0.5 \text{ g} = 1 \times \frac{\overset{2}{\cancel{10}}}{\cancel{5}} = 2$$

Therefore two tablets, gr $7\frac{1}{2}$ (0.5 g), are needed to make 1000 ml of 1 : 1000 solution.

FINDING THE AMOUNT OF SOLUTION THAT CAN BE PREPARED FROM A KNOWN QUANTITY OF DRUG

In the previous problems the unknown factor was the solute. In the following problems the total amount of solution is unknown.

Problem 1

How much 2% solution can be prepared from 10 ml of pure drug?

Analyzing the problem reveals the following factors:

$$\begin{aligned} 2\% &= \text{strength desired} \\ 100\% &= \text{strength on hand} \\ 10 \text{ ml} &= \text{amount of solute} \\ x &= \text{total amount of solution} \end{aligned}$$

The strengths of the solutions are in like terms. The solute is in milliliters, and the total amount of solution will be expressed in milliliters. Conversions are not needed. The unknown term is the quantity of solution and can be solved as follows:

$$\frac{2\% \text{ strength desired}}{100\% \text{ strength on hand}} \times x \text{ quantity of solution} = 10 \text{ ml, amount of solute}$$

Simplify:

$$\frac{2\%}{100\%} = \frac{1}{50}$$

$$\frac{1}{50}x = 10$$

$$x = 10 \div \frac{1}{50} = 10 \times \frac{50}{1} = 500$$

$$x = 500$$

$\therefore$ 500 ml is the total amount of solution.

To make the solution add a quantity of water to 10 ml of pure drug to make 500 ml. This is 490 ml.

Proof: When x is the quantity of solution, proof is obtained by the product multiplied by the divisor; the result equals the dividend.

Problem 2

How much ½% solution can be made from 2 g?

Analyzing the problem reveals the following factors:

$$\begin{aligned} \tfrac{1}{2}\% &= \text{strength desired} \\ 100\% &= \text{strength on hand} \\ 2 \text{ g} &= \text{amount of solute} \\ x &= \text{total amount of solution} \end{aligned}$$

No conversions need to be made since the strengths of the solutions are in like terms. The solute is in grams so that the problem will be worked in the metric system and the answer will be expressed in milliliters. The problem will read as follows:

$$\frac{\tfrac{1}{2}\% \text{ strength desired}}{100\% \text{ strength on hand}} \times x \text{ quantity of solution} = 2 \text{ g, amount of solute}$$

Simplify:

$$\frac{\frac{1}{2}\%}{100\%} = \frac{0.1}{20}$$

$$\frac{0.1}{20}x = 2$$

$$x = 2 \div \frac{0.1}{20} = 2 \times \frac{20}{0.1} = 400$$

$$x = 400$$

∴ 400 ml of ½% solution can be made from 2 g.

Proof: $\overset{4}{\cancel{400}} \times \frac{0.5}{\cancel{100}} = 2$

Problem 3

How much 1:500 solution can be made from a gr 15 tablet?
Analyzing the problem, the factors are as follows:

1:500 = strength desired
100% = strength on hand
gr 15 = solute
x = quantity of solution

The strengths of the solutions are unlike and will need to be converted to like terms, either percent to percent or ratio to ratio. The drug on hand is in grains. This would indicate that the problem should be solved in the apothecaries' system, and the answer would be in ounces, drams, or minims. However, the student should recognize immediately that gr 15 equal 1 g; therefore it is best to solve in the metric system to get a practical measurement. Changing the ratio strength of the solution desired to % is 0.2%. The problem will read as follows:

$$\frac{0.2\% \text{ strength desired}}{100\% \text{ strength on hand}} \times x = 1 \text{ g}$$

Simplify:

$$\frac{0.2\%}{100\%} = \frac{1}{500}$$

$$\frac{1}{500}x = 1$$

$$x = 1 \div \frac{1}{500} = 1 \times \frac{500}{1} = 500$$

$$x = 500$$

∴ 500 ml solution can be made.

$$\text{Proof: } \overset{1}{\cancel{500}} \times \frac{1}{\cancel{500}} = 1$$

Solutions from stock solutions

Stock solutions are relatively strong solutions from which weaker solutions are made. These solutions may be labeled in percent, ratio, or the amount of drug in the solution.

In the preceding problems solutions were prepared from full-strength solutions and drugs (100%). In stock solutions the drug is already in a solution of given strength of less than 100%. These solutions are used to make weaker solutions of a desired strength. The same methods are used in preparing solutions from stock solutions as from full-strength drugs. However, it is very important to remember that the strengths of stock solutions are less than full-strength solutions.

FINDING THE AMOUNT OF STOCK SOLUTION NEEDED TO PREPARE A GIVEN AMOUNT OF SOLUTION OF DESIRED STRENGTH

Problem

Prepare 1 liter of 2% solution from a 40% solution. How much stock solution is required?

Analyzing the problem shows the following factors:

$$\begin{aligned} 2\% &= \text{strength desired} \\ 40\% &= \text{strength on hand} \\ x &= \text{solute} \\ 1 \text{ liter} &= \text{total amount of solution} \end{aligned}$$

The unknown quantity is the solute. The strengths are in like terms. The quantity is in liters and will have to be changed to milliliters. The answer to the problem will be in milliliters.

Using the rule

$$\frac{\text{strength desired}}{\text{strength on hand}} \times \text{quantity of solution} = \text{amount of solute}$$

the problem reads as follows:

$$\frac{2\% \text{ strength desired}}{40\% \text{ strength on hand}} \times 1000 = x$$

Simplify:

$$\frac{2\%}{40\%} = \frac{1}{20}$$

$$\frac{1}{\cancel{20}} \times \overset{50}{\cancel{1000}} = x$$

$$x = 50$$

∴ 50 ml of stock solution is needed.

Proof: The product divided by the multiplier equals the multiplicand.

$$50 \div 1000 = \cancel{50} \times \frac{1}{\underset{20}{\cancel{1000}}} = \frac{1}{20}$$

To prepare the solution add sufficient water to 50 ml of 40% stock solution to make 1000 ml.

PREPARING AN UNKNOWN QUANTITY OF SOLUTION OF DESIRED STRENGTH FROM STOCK SOLUTION

Problem

How much 1:50 boric acid solution can be prepared from 1 ℥ of 1:20 boric acid solution?

Analyzing the problem reveals the following:

1:50 = strength desired
1:20 = strength on hand
1 ℥ = amount of solute
x = total amount of solution

The strengths of the solutions are in like terms. The problem can be worked in the metric or apothecaries' system. Solving in the apothecaries' system, the equation will read as follows:

$$\frac{1/50 \text{ strength desired}}{1/20 \text{ strength on hand}} \times x = 1$$

Simplify:

$$\frac{1/50}{1/20} = \frac{2}{5}$$

$$\frac{2}{5}x = 1$$

$$x = 1 \times \frac{5}{2} = 2\tfrac{1}{2}$$

$$x = 2\tfrac{1}{2}$$

$\therefore$ 1 ℥ of 1:20 solution will make 2½ ℥ 1:50 solution.

Add sufficient water (1½ ℥) to 1 ℥ of 1:20 solution to make 2½ ℥ of 1:50 solution.

Proof: The product multiplied by the divisor equals the dividend.

$$2\tfrac{1}{2} \times \tfrac{2}{5} = \frac{\overset{1}{\cancel{5}}}{\cancel{2}} \times \frac{\overset{1}{\cancel{2}}}{\cancel{5}} = 1$$

Determining the percentage or ratio strength of solutions

Orders requiring the use of solutions most often express the strength in percent or ratio. However, some stock solutions are labeled indicating the amount of drug dissolved in a specified amount of solution. This makes it necessary to find the strength of the solution expressed in percent or ratio when (1) the strength of the solution is expressed by the amount of drug (solute) to a given quantity of solution or (2) the strength of the solution is expressed by a ratio.

Any of the mathematical processes previously employed can be used to find the percentage strength of solutions: by simple arithmetic, what percent one number is of another; by proportion by finding the missing factor; and by the formula

$$\frac{\%\text{ desired}}{\%\text{ on hand}} \times \text{quantity} = \text{solute}$$

when *% desired* is the missing factor.

Simple arithmetic is the most direct method. It saves time and reduces the chance for error.

FINDING THE PERCENTAGE STRENGTH OF A SOLUTION

Problem 1

One-half liter of sodium chloride solution contains 1 dram of sodium chloride. What is the percentage strength?

Analyzing the problem: The liter will have to be changed to milliliters.
The dram will have to be changed to milliliters or grams.

1. If solved by arithmetic, the problem reads as follows: What % of 500 is 4 g? (Refer to p. 33 if necessary.)

$$\frac{4}{500} = 4 \div 500 = 500\overline{)4.000} \quad 0.008 = 0.8\%$$

0.008 × 100 moves the decimal point two places to the right and gives 0.8%.

2. If solved by proportion, the factors are as follows:

$$x = \text{unknown \% strength}$$
$$100\% = \text{full strength}$$

$$4 \text{ g} = \text{amount of solute}$$
$$500 \text{ ml} = \text{total amount of solution}$$

$$x:100 = 4:500$$
$$500x = 400$$
$$x = 400 \div 500 = \overset{4}{\cancel{400}} \times \frac{1}{\underset{5}{\cancel{500}}} = \frac{4}{5}$$
$$x = 4/5 \text{ or } 0.8\%$$

3. If the problem is solved by the formula

$$\frac{\% \text{ desired}}{\% \text{ on hand}} \times \text{quantity} = \text{solute}$$

% desired is the unknown factor.

$$\frac{x}{100\%} \times 500 = 4$$
$$\frac{x}{1} \times 500 = 4$$
$$x = 4 \div 500 = \cancel{4} \times \frac{1}{\underset{125}{\cancel{500}}} = \frac{1}{125} \text{ or } 0.008$$
$$x = 0.008 \text{ or } 0.8\%$$

Problem 2

What is the percentage strength of a solution in a bottle labeled 1:20?

When the strength of a solution is expressed as a ratio, the percentage strength can be found by a simple rule.

Rule: To change a ratio to percent, express the ratio as a common fraction, divide the numerator by the denominator and multiply by 100. Add the % sign.

$$1:20 = \frac{1}{20}$$

$$20\overline{)1.00} = 0.05 \qquad 0.05 \times 100 = 5\%$$

Multiplying by 100 moves the decimal point two places to the right.

FINDING RATIO STRENGTH OF A SOLUTION

To find the ratio strength of a solution when

1. The strength of the solution is expressed by the amount of drug (solute) to a given quantity of solution.
2. The strength is expressed as a percent.

Problem 1

One liter of solution contains 50 ml of pure drug. What is the ratio strength?

The simplest way to obtain the ratio strength is to express the relationship of solute to solution as a fraction (reduce fraction to its lowest terms, if necessary). The numerator of the fraction will be the first term of the ratio and the denominator, the second term.

Solute : solution expressed as a fraction is $^{50}/_{1000}$

$^{50}/_{1000}$ reduced to lowest terms = $^{1}/_{20}$

$^{1}/_{20}$ expressed as a ratio is 1:20

Problem 2

What is the ratio strength of a solution labeled 20%?

The ratio strength is quickly found by changing the percent to a fraction (reduce to lowest terms, if necessary) and expressing the fraction as a ratio.

20% = $^{20}/_{100}$ reduced to lowest terms = $^{1}/_{5}$

$^{1}/_{5}$ expressed as a ratio is 1:5

PROBLEMS

Name ______________________

Date ______________________

EXTERNAL DOSAGE

Solutions from pure or full-strength drugs

In these problems the amount of solute, the amount of solvent, or the amount of solution is unknown. All drugs used are pure or full-strength drugs. Answers must be labeled.

In making relatively large quantities of solution for external use, a fraction of a milliliter less than one half is dropped; for a fraction of $\frac{1}{2}$ ml or more, the next higher whole number is used.

EXAMPLE: $1\frac{1}{4}$ ml would be measured as 1 ml, $1\frac{1}{2}$ ml or $1\frac{3}{4}$ ml would be measured as 2 ml.

1. How much physiologic (0.9%) saline solution can be made from 9 g of salt?

____

2. How many ounces of iodine crystals are needed to make 450 ml of 7% solution?

____

3. How much 1:5000 potassium permanganate can be made from 100 mg?

____

4. How much alcohol is needed to make 1000 ml of 70% solution?

____

5. How much cocaine is in ♏ 250 of 2% solution?

____

6. How much water will need to be added to 100 ml of 100% alcohol to make a 20% solution?

____

7. How much 1% silver nitrate can be made from 1 g of crystals?

____

8. How much 1% neomycin sulfate solution can be made from 5 g?

____

9. How much table salt is needed to make a quart of physiologic (0.9%) saline solution? How much is this in household measure?

____

10. How much soda bicarbonate powder is needed to prepare 400 ml of 2% solution for mouthwash? How much is this in household measure?

____

PROBLEMS

Name ______________________

Date ______________________

EXTERNAL DOSAGE—cont'd
Solutions from stock solutions

Find the amount of stock solution required, diluent required, or total solution that can be made. Answers must be labeled. A fraction of a milliliter should be rounded off to the nearest whole number.

1. How much 1% solution can be made from 4 ml of 5% stock solution?

   ____

2. How much 70% alcohol solution is needed to prepare 280 ml of 25% solution?

   ____

3. There is a 5-ml ampule of 10% solution on hand. How much 0.1% solution can be made?

   ____

4. How much 1% atropine sulfate solution is needed to prepare ½ ℥ of ½% solution?

   ____

5. How much 7% iodine is needed to make 175 ml of 2% solution?

   ____

6. There is 100 ml of a 1:1000 solution on hand. How much 1:5000 solution can be made from it?

____

7. The available sterile saline solution is 60 ml of 10% strength. The physician requires a 3% solution. How much diluent is needed?

____

8. How much 5% boric acid solution is needed to prepare 500 ml of 2% solution?

____

9. How much 0.45% saline solution is needed to prepare a liter of 0.2% saline solution?

____

10. There is 200 ml of a 3% hydrogen peroxide on hand. How much 1% solution of hydrogen peroxide can be made?

____

PROBLEMS

Name ______________________

Date ______________________

EXTERNAL DOSAGE—cont'd

Percentage strength of solutions

What is the percentage strength of the following solutions?

1. a. 3:250 solution ____________
   b. 1:4000 solution ____________
   c. 1:5 solution ____________
   d. 2:3 solution ____________
   e. 2:25 solution ____________
   f. $\frac{7}{200}$ solution ____________
   g. $\frac{1}{10}$ solution ____________
   h. $\frac{1}{2}$ solution ____________
   i. $\frac{8}{5}$ solution ____________
   j. $\frac{1}{1000}$ solution ____________

2. 400 g in 1 gallon of saline solution?

   ____

3. A solution containing 1 g to $\frac{1}{2}$ liter?

   ____

4. Gr 15 of potassium permanganate in 1 liter of water?

   ____

5. $\frac{1}{4}$ liter of alcohol in 1 liter of solution?

   ____

What is the percentage strength of the following solutions?—cont'd

6. 4 ml of lidocaine solution containing 0.5 g of lidocaine? __________

7. 0.05 g of polymyxin B in 500 ml of solution? __________

8. 1 gallon of solution containing 20 g of the drug? __________

9. 30 g in 400 ml of solution? __________

10. 8 g of boric acid crystals in ½ liter of solution? __________

PROBLEMS

Name ______________________

Date ______________________

EXTERNAL DOSAGE—cont'd
Ratio strength of solutions

What is the ratio strength of the following solutions?

1. a. 15% solution ____________ f. 12% solution ____________

   b. 70% solution ____________ g. $33\frac{1}{3}$% solution ____________

   c. 0.9% solution ____________ h. 3% solution ____________

   d. 125% solution ____________ i. 0.1% solution ____________

   e. 100% solution ____________ j. 0.4% solution ____________

2. 180 ml of boric acid solution that contains 30 g of crystals?

   ____

3. 60 ml of Merthiolate solution that contains 0.4 g of crystals?

   ____

4. 600 ml of potassium permanganate solution that contains 0.3 g?

   ____

5. 100 ml of solution containing 0.6 g of drug?

   ____

What is the ratio strength of the following solutions?—cont'd

6. 800 ml of solution containing 0.5 g of drug?

____

7. 1800 ml of solution that contains 3 g of drug?

____

8. 750 ml of solution that contains 30 ml of drug?

____

9. 1 gal of saline solution that contains gr 60 of salt?

____

10. 2000 ml of solution that contains 60 g of drug?

____

CHAPTER 11

Oral Dosage

OBJECTIVES

At the completion of this chapter, the student will:

- calculate oral dosage from stock solutions
- calculate oral dosage from tablets and capsules

The most common method for the administration of drugs is orally. Generally this method is a safe, convenient, and effective way to administer drugs for local and systemic effect. Absorption of the drug takes place in the gastrointestinal tract. Drugs for oral administration may be in the form of liquids, solids, and powders.

Computation of the dosage of drugs administered orally may be necessary because

1. The drug in stock is expressed in a different measure than that of the drug ordered.
2. The dose of the drug in stock may be larger or smaller than the dose ordered.
3. The amount of drug in solution is expressed as a percentage or as a stated amount in a given unit of measure.

The strength of drugs is usually measured in the metric system and the apothecaries' system. However, the apothecaries' system has limited use. The dosage of some drugs is measured in ''units.'' U is the abbreviation for units. The strength of a drug expressed in units varies from drug to drug and is indicated on the label.

ORAL DOSAGE OF DRUGS IN SOLUTION

Drugs in solution are prepared commercially or in the pharmacy and contain a specific amount of drug in a given amount of solution as stated on the label. The required dosage is computed from the information on the label. When the dosage desired and the dosage on hand (as indicated on the label) are not in the same units of measurement, they must be converted to the same units.

EXAMPLES:

1. Morphine sulfate elixir is labeled 10 mg in 5 ml. How much will be needed to give 15 mg?

   The simple method to use is as follows:

$$\frac{\text{dose desired}}{\text{dose on hand}} \times \text{quantity} = \text{amount to give}$$

$$\frac{15\ \text{mg}}{10\ \text{mg}} \times 5\ \text{ml} = x\ \text{ml}$$

$$\frac{15}{10} \times 5 = 7\tfrac{1}{2}$$

∴ 7½ ml is needed to give 15 mg.

When the quantity is 1, as in this problem, it is not necessary to show the (× quantity) step. The abbreviated equation is written as $\frac{D}{H} = x$.

2. Potassium chloride solution is labeled 30%. Give 0.6 g.

   The drug desired and the drug on hand must be converted to the same unit of measure. Changing 30% to grams equals 0.3 g in 1 ml.

$$\frac{D}{H} = x$$

$$\frac{0.3}{0.6} = x$$

$$x = \frac{6}{10} \div \frac{3}{10} = \frac{\overset{2}{\cancel{6}}}{\underset{1}{\cancel{10}}} \times \frac{\overset{1}{\cancel{10}}}{\underset{1}{\cancel{3}}} = 2$$

$$x = 2$$

∴ 2 ml of 30% solution is needed to give 0.6 g. Give ♏ 32.

Observe that there are 0.3 g in 1 ml. To give 0.6 g, 2 × 0.3 g, or 2 ml, is needed. Therefore the mathematical procedure is not needed in this problem.

In the oral administration of a drug, a fraction less than ♏ ½ is dropped; if a fraction is ♏ ½ or more, the next highest whole number is used.

An amount of liquid as small as 2 ml is difficult to give and should be diluted with a convenient amount of water unless contraindicated. To measure dosages of this amount, oral liquid dispensers arc available in sizes of 1 ml, 5 ml, and 10 ml with teaspoon, fractional teaspoon, and milliliter calibrations. The dispenser provides syringe-like accuracy.

ORAL DOSAGE FROM DRUGS IN SOLID FORM

Drugs in solid form come in the strength of the dose or doses in which they are commonly used. It is always desirable to obtain the drug in the strength of the desired dose or a multiple of the desired dose. Because pills, tablets, and capsules cannot be accurately divided, tablets of a large dose are not recommended for the preparation of a smaller dose in oral administration.

Computing oral dosage of drugs in tablet and capsule form requires accurate conversion of measure from the apothecaries' system to the metric system and vice versa and finding the number of tablets or capsules to give.

To find the desired dose, use $\frac{D}{H} = x$.

EXAMPLES:

1. Codeine sulfate 30 mg is on hand. How many tablets are needed to give gr 1?

The dose desired and the dose on hand are not in the same system of measures; both will have to be in milligrams or grams. In the apothecaries' system 30 mg equals gr ½. Solve the problem as follows:

$$\frac{1}{1/2} = x$$

$$x = 1 \div \frac{1}{2} = 1 \times \frac{2}{1}$$

$$x = 2$$

∴ 2 tablets are needed to give gr 1.

2. Penicillin VK is available in 400,000 U tablets. How many tablets are required to give a total daily dose of 1,600,000 U?

It can be seen that four tablets are needed. Many of these problems will not require an arithmetic procedure. However, it is important that the terms in the problem are in the same unit of measure and that when necessary the correct conversion is made.

3. Zyloprim is available in 100-mg and 300-mg tablets; gr 1½ is ordered three times a day. How many tablets are needed for each dose? What strength? Convert gr 1½ to 100 mg.

   ∴ one 100 mg tablet is needed for each dose three times a day.

ORAL DOSAGE FROM DRUGS IN POWDER FORM

Drugs in powder form come from the pharmacy weighed, packeted in individual doses, and labeled for a specific patient. The nurse is seldom asked to give a fractional dose from a packet but should know what to do if the situation arises.

EXAMPLES:

1. A packet contains 500 mg of drug. Give 125 mg. Prepare a solution by dissolving the drug in a desirable amount of water. How much of the solution is needed to give 125 mg? Dissolve 500 mg in 30 ml of water.

$$\frac{125}{500} = x$$

$$x = 125 \div 500 = 0.25$$

$$x = 0.25 \text{ or } 1/4$$

$$1/4 \text{ of } 30 \text{ ml} = 7\tfrac{1}{2} \text{ or } 8 \text{ ml } (2\ ʒ)$$

∴ 8 ml (2 ʒ) are needed to give 125 mg.

2. A packet contains 4 g of drug. Give 1.5 g. Prepare a solution by dissolving the drug in a desirable amount of liquid. How much of the solution is needed to give 1.5 g? Dissolve 4 g in 120 ml of fruit juice.

$$\frac{1.5}{4} = x$$

$$x = 1.5 \div 4 = 0.375$$

$$x = 0.375$$

$$0.375 \text{ of } 120 \text{ ml} = 45 \text{ ml } (1\tfrac{1}{2} \text{ oz.})$$

$\therefore$ 45 ml (1½ oz.) are needed to give 1.5 g.

MEASUREMENT OF DOSAGE IN MINIMS

Medicines ordered in minims for oral administration must be measured in a minim graduate or calibrated syringe. A medicine dropper is not accurate for measuring minims.

The minim graduate is calibrated to 60 ♏ in multiples of five. When the amount of drug needed is not in a multiple of five, there is a simple procedure to use to measure the odd minims.

PROCEDURE: Pour 5 ♏ of drug in a minim graduate. Dilute five times. (5 × 5 = 25 ♏ of a 1:5 solution.) 5 ♏ of the new solution contains 1 ♏ of the original drug. Discard the amount of new solution not needed. To the remainder add the number of minims that are measurable by a multiple of five. If the student wishes, the minims in multiples of five can be measured first and poured into a medicine graduate and then odd minims can be measured.

PROBLEM: Prepare ♏ 28 of a drug. What is the total amount of solution?

1. Prepare ♏ 25 of 1:5 solution. (♏ 5 of the new solution contains ♏ 1 of the original drug.) (Fig. 2, *A*.)
2. Measure number of minims needed. (3 × 5 = ♏ 15 of the 1:5 solution is needed.)

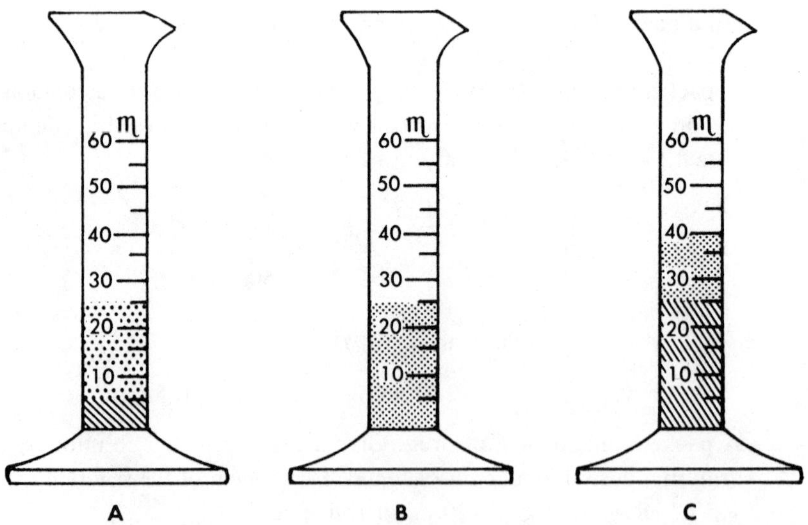

Fig. 2

3. Discard ♏ 10.
4. To ♏ 15 add ♏ 25 (Fig. 2, *B*) of the undiluted drug.
5. ♏ 15 + ♏ 25 = ♏ 40, the total amount of solution in which there is ♏ 28 of the original drug (Fig. 2, *C*).

PROBLEMS

Name ______________________

Date ______________________

ORAL DOSAGE

Oral dosage from stock solutions

Answers must be labeled.

1. Tetracycline syrup 2 g in a 2-ounce bottle; 125 mg ordered.

   ____

2. Elixir terpin hydrate with codeine has gr ⅛ codeine in 1 tsp; how much codeine would be administered if 1 tsp were given every 4 hours for a total of 6 doses?

   ____

3. Dilaudid hydrochloride solution 2 mg in 1 ml; 2.5 mg is ordered.

   ____

4. Methadone elixir 5 mg in 5 ml; 12 mg is ordered.

   ____

5. Robitussin cough syrup 600 mg in 1 ounce; 225 mg is ordered.

   ____

6. Potassium chloride 10%; gr viiss ordered.

____

7. Ferrous sulfate 2 g in fl ℥ i; gr v ordered.

____

8. Elixir phenobarbital contains 4 mg of drug in 1 ml; fl ʒ i is ordered.

____

9. Ferrous sulfate 40 mg in 1 ml; 240 mg ordered.

____

10. Elixir acetaminophen 120 mg in 5 ml; gr v ordered.

____

11. Benzathine penicillin G in 2-ounce bottles; one contains 300,000 U in 5 ml, the other 500,000 U in 5 ml; give 400,000 U. (a) Using bottle 1, how much is needed; (b) bottle 2, how much is needed?

a. ______________; b. ______________

PROBLEMS

Name ____________________

Date ____________________

ORAL DOSAGE—cont'd

12. A solution contains 500 μg of drug in one dram; 750 μg is ordered.

____

13. Haldol concentrate 2 mg per 1 ml; 0.5 mg is ordered.

____

14. Thorazine concentrate 100 mg in 1 ml; 325 mg is ordered.

____

15. Erythromycin ethylsuccinate suspension 200 mg in 5 ml. Dosage is 50 mg/kg body weight/day, and the person weighs 88 pounds. (a) What is the total daily dosage? (b) What is the individual dose if the drug is given q. 6 h.? Determine dosage in mg and ml.

a. ____________ mg; ____________ ml

b. ____________ mg; ____________ ml

Oral dosage from tablets and capsules

Give the number of tablets or capsules needed.

1. Orinase, 500-mg tablets. Give 1 g after breakfast, 0.5 g after lunch and dinner. How many tablets are given after each meal?

   a. Breakfast ________; b. Lunch ________; c. Dinner ________

2. Atropine sulfate gr $^{1}/_{300}$ tablets. Give gr $^{1}/_{150}$.

   ____

3. Hydrodiuril 50-mg tablets. Give gr $1\,^{1}/_{2}$.

   ____

4. Dilantin 100-mg capsules. Give 0.3 g.

   ____

5. Gantrisin 0.5-g tablets. Give gr xv.

   ____

PROBLEMS

Name ____________________

Date ____________________

ORAL DOSAGE—cont'd

6. Tegretol 0.2-g tablets. Give gr vi q.i.d. How many tablets for each dose?

   ____

7. Codeine sulfate 15-mg tablets. Give (a) gr ss; (b) gr $\frac{1}{4}$.

   a. ____________; b. ____________

8. Prednisone 5-mg and 10-mg tablets. Give gr $\frac{1}{4}$ daily. (a) What size tablets should be used? (b) How many?

   a. ____________; b. ____________

9. Levothyroxin 100 μg tablets. Give gr $\frac{1}{300}$.

   ____

10. Tagamet 300-mg tablets. Give 1.2 g daily in four divided doses. How many tablets will the patient take per day?

   ____

11. Pyridoxine hydrochloride 10-mg and 25-mg tablets. Give gr ½. (a) What size tablet should be used? (b) How many?

a. ______________; b. ______________

12. Phenergan hydrochloride 12.5-mg tablets. Give 25 mg.

____

13. Neomycin tablets 0.5 g available. Dosage is 0.06 g/kg of body weight per day. If a person weighs 154 lb, (a) what is the total daily dosage, (b) what is the individual q.i.d. dose, and (c) how many tablets are used for each dose?

a. ______________; b. ______________; c. ______________

14. Erythromycin 2 g daily, divided into four doses. How many grams in each dose?

____

15. Keflex is available in 0.25-g capsules. 0.5 g is ordered q.i.d. How many capsules are needed daily?

____

PROBLEMS

Name ____________________

Date ____________________

ORAL DOSAGE—cont'd

16. Procainamide 1 g is ordered as an initial dose and 0.5 g q.i.d. thereafter. 500-mg capsules are available. How many capsules are needed for (a) initial dose and (b) daily dose?

a. ____________; b. ____________

17. Erythromycin, amoxicillin, and chloramphenicol are available in 250-mg capsules. How many capsules are needed to give the following:

a. 0.5 g ____________; b. 0.75 g ____________; c. gr viiss ____________

18. On hand is tetracycline 100-mg, 250-mg, and 500-mg capsules. Give 1 g in four equal doses at 6-hour intervals. (a) How many milligrams in each dose? (b) What size capsules will you use?

a. ____________; b. ____________

19. Doxepin hydrochloride 10-mg capsules. Give gr ½.

____

20. Thyroid gr ii. Give 120 mg.

____

21. Phenobarbital gr 1½ tablets. Give 0.05 g.

____

22. Clonopin 0.5-mg tablets. Dosage is 0.1 mg/kg body weight, and the person weighs 110 pounds. (a) What is the total daily dosage? (b) What is the individual dose if the drug is given q.i.d.?

a. _______________; b. _______________

23. Theo-Dur is available in 100-mg, 200-mg, and 300-mg sustained action tablets. In order to obtain a serum theophylline concentration between 10 and 20 μg/ml, an adult weighing 165 pounds requires a dose of 8 mg/kg body weight. (a) What is the total daily dose? (b) What is the individual dose if the drug is given q. 12 h.?

a. _______________; b. _______________

24. Procainamide is available in 250-mg, 375-mg, and 500-mg tablets. The dosage is 50 mg/kg body weight daily given in divided doses at 4-hour intervals. (a) What is the total daily dose for an adult weighing 132 pounds? (b) What is the individual dose?

a. _______________; b. _______________

25. Antepar tablets 500 mg. Give 3.5 g.

____

CHAPTER 12

Parenteral Dosage

OBJECTIVES

At the completion of this chapter, the student will:

- calculate parenteral dosage of drugs from stock on hand in vials or ampules
- measure correct units of insulin in appropriate syringe
- calculate doses of intravenous fluids and electrolytes
- determine flow rates of intravenous solution
- determine dosage of hyperalimentation rates

Parenteral administration of drugs is the injection of drugs into the tissues by needle.

Advantages of this method

1. Rapid action of drug.
2. Can be used when drug cannot be given by mouth.
3. The therapeutic dose can be accurately gauged since the drug is absorbed directly into the bloodstream.

Injection of drugs may be given

1. Intradermally—into the upper layers of the skin.
2. Subcutaneously—into the loose tissues beneath the skin. This is known as hypodermic injection.
3. Intramuscularly—into the underlying muscles, usually the buttocks. Drugs that are irritating are given in this manner.
4. Intravenously—given directly into the vein.
5. Intraspinally—given directly into the subarachnoid space of the spinal cord.

In most hospitals nurses have the responsibility of administering intradermal, subcutaneous, and intramuscular drugs. Specially trained nurses or physicians administer intravenous solutions. Only physicians administer drugs intraspinally.

Relatively small amounts of solution are injected parenterally except when the intravenous route is utilized. Large amounts of solution given intravenously are called infusions.

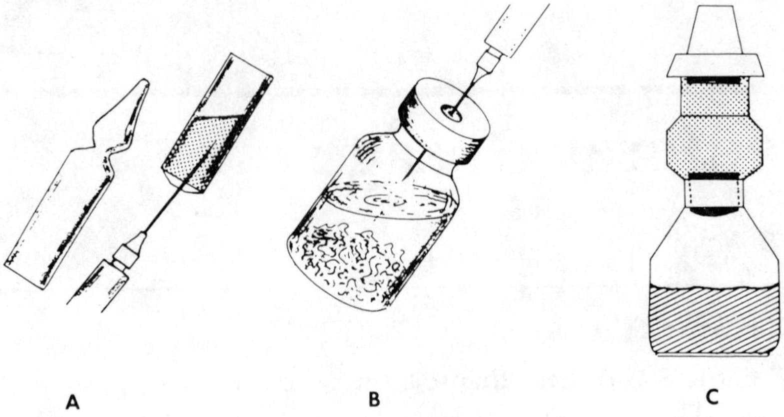

Fig. 3. A, Ampule, **B,** Instilling diluent into vial with drug in dry form. **C,** Individual dose vial containing a diluent and dry drug.

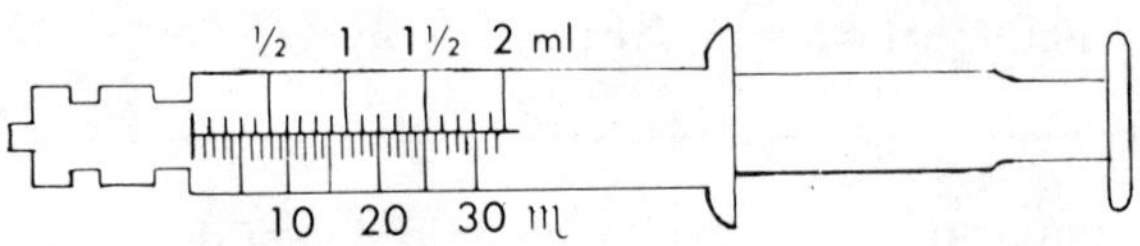

Fig. 4. Standard 2-ml hypodermic syringe.

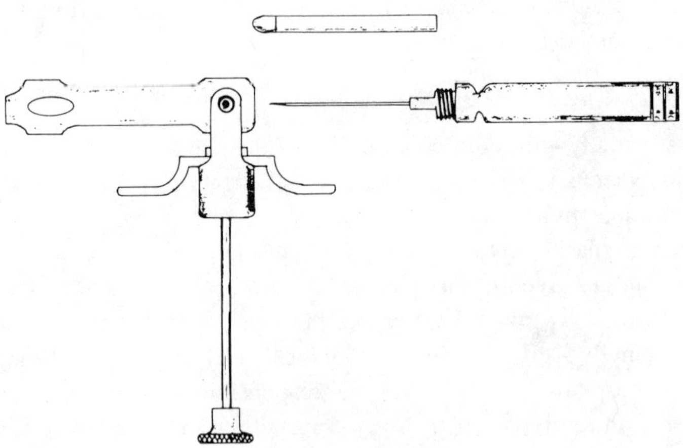

Fig. 5. Metal syringe with disposable cartridge and needle unit.

Preparations of drugs for injection come in various forms

1. *Ampules* are sealed glass containers usually containing one dose of the drug (Fig. 3, *A*). The ampule is broken at the neck to insert the needle and withdraw the drug into the hypodermic syringe (Fig. 4).
2. *Vials* are glass containers with rubber stoppers usually containing multiple doses of the drug (Fig. 3, *B*). The needle is inserted through the rubber stopper of the vial and the desired dose is withdrawn.

   Ampules and vials contain drugs in either liquid or powder form. Drugs that deteriorate in solution come in the dry state, and the diluent is added when the drug is to be administered. Some unstable drugs come in a single-dose unit containing the drug and the solvent in separate compartments (Fig. 3, *C*). Pressure on top of the unit releases the rubber plug between the compartments, and the drug is dissolved.
3. *Prefilled disposable syringe units* for the administration of drugs by injection are also on the market. The entire unit may be disposable or only a part, such as a cartridge containing the drug. These units are usually calibrated and contain a definite amount of drug in a specified volume (Fig. 5).

DOSAGE OF DRUGS FROM STOCK SOLUTION

Stock solutions come in rubber-stoppered vials containing multiple doses. The strength of the solution is expressed in percentage, ratio, or a stated amount of drug in 1 ml.

Problems

1. Give morphine sulfate gr 1/8 from a stock solution containing gr 1/4 per milliliter. How much stock solution is needed?

$$\frac{D}{H} = x \text{ (amount of solution needed)}$$

$$\frac{1/8}{1/4} = \frac{1}{\underset{2}{\cancel{8}}} \times \frac{\cancel{4}}{1} = \frac{1}{2}$$

∴ 1/2 ml (♏ 8) is needed to give gr 1/8.

2. Prepare mannitol 1 g from a 25% stock solution. How much 25% solution is needed?

25% changed to a fraction and reduced is 1/4

$$\frac{D}{H} = x \text{ (amount of solution needed)}$$

$$\frac{1}{1/4} = 1 \times \frac{4}{1} = 4$$

∴ 4 ml of 25% solution is needed.

3. Give Levo-Dromoran gr $\frac{1}{20}$ from a 10-ml vial labeled 2 mg/ml. The drug must be in like terms. Changing gr $\frac{1}{20}$ to mg equals 3 mg.

$$\frac{D}{H} = x \text{ (amount of solution needed)}$$

$$\frac{3}{2} = 1\frac{1}{2}$$

$\therefore 1\frac{1}{2}$ ml is needed to give 3 mg.

DOSAGE FROM DRUGS IN DRY FORM

The amount of drug in a vial may contain the exact dose or multiple doses. In either case, sterile diluent must be added before the drug can be administered. The common diluent is sterile distilled water. In a single-dose vial add the amount of diluent stated on the vial, or use 1 ml to 1.5 ml for intramuscular injection. In a multiple-dose vial it is desirable to dissolve the drug in the amount of diluent necessary to make 1 ml equal the desired dose. Vials for multiple doses usually have a capacity of 10 ml and 20 ml. The volume of the powder is not considered to contribute significantly to the volume of the solution *unless* otherwise indicated by the manufacturer's directions for mixing the solution. Therefore the quantity of diluent may be considered in most cases to be the volume of the final solution. However, lyophilized powders do occupy a certain volume in solution. If this volume is not taken into account, the wrong amount of diluent will be added to the drug, and the wrong dose may be administered to the patient. After diluting a multidose vial, label the vial with the amount of diluent used and the concentration of drug per milliliter of solution.

EXAMPLES:

1. Sodium cephalothin (Keflin) is supplied in a vial containing 1 g. The manufacturer's directions say to prepare a 1-g solution, add 4 ml of diluent. This will provide 0.5 g in 2.2 ml of solution. Therefore the volume of powder in the vial is equivalent to 0.4 ml of solution.

How much of the solution prepared according to the manufacturer's directions would be needed for a 0.25 g dose of sodium cephalothin (Keflin)?

$$2.2 \text{ ml} = 0.5 \text{ g}$$

$$\frac{0.25}{0.5} = x$$

$$x = \frac{1}{2}$$

$$\frac{1}{2} \text{ of } 2.2 = 1.1 \text{ ml } (♏ 17)$$

$\therefore$ 1.1 ml (♏ 17) is needed to give 0.25 g of drug.

2. A vial contains 5,000,000 U of penicillin in dry form. A solution is needed that contains 500,000 U in 1 ml. The manufacturer's directions for this particular brand and amount of penicillin indicate to prepare a solution with a concentration of 500,000 U/ml, add 8 ml of diluent. There are ten 500,000 U doses in the

vial containing 5,000,000 U. Therefore the total volume in the vial must be 10 ml and the manufacturer is inferring that the powder volume is 2 ml.

$$\frac{5{,}000{,}000}{500{,}000} = 10 \text{ doses of } 500{,}000 \text{ U/ml.}$$

8 ml diluent added plus 2 ml powder volume equals 10 ml.

How much of this solution is needed to give 800,000 U?

The total amount of solution is the unknown quantity and is found by the following formula:

$$\frac{D}{H} = x$$

$$\frac{800{,}000 \text{ units}}{500{,}000 \text{ units}} = \frac{8}{5}$$

$$8/5 = 1\,3/5$$

$\therefore$ 1 3/5 ml of 500,000 U/ml solution is needed.

3. A 2-ml ampule contains 0.5 g dry drug. No directions for mixing the solution are given by the manufacturer. Therefore the quantity of diluent added may be considered to be the volume of the final solution. A dose of 200 mg is needed. How many milliliters are needed?

Step 1. Dissolve 0.5 g by injecting 2 ml of sterile distilled water into the ampule. This gives a solution containing 0.5 g in 2 ml.

Step 2. Change 0.5 g to mg = 500 mg

$$\frac{200}{500} = \frac{2}{5}$$

2/5 of 2 ml is needed

2/5 of 2 ml = 4/5 ml (♏12)

$\therefore$ 4/5 ml (♏12) is needed to give 200 mg.

DOSAGE OF INSULIN

The U.S.P. standardization of insulin is in units. Originally the unit of insulin was based on the hypoglycemic effect in rabbits. Now a unit is based on an absolute weight of insulin prepared from a recrystallized composite sample. Insulin is used in the treatment of diabetes mellitus.

Insulin is supplied in rubber-stoppered, multidose vials of 10 ml. The strengths most commonly used are 40 or 100 U/ml designated as U 40 and U 100. Each strength of insulin is identified by the color of the "flip-off" cap. Red identifies U 40; and orange U 100. Regular insulin (concentrated) containing 500 U/ml is available for use in cases of insulin resistance in which patients require very high doses.

U 100 insulin was introduced to standardize the concentration of insulin available to all diabetic persons. Health professionals should be aware that a complete move to insulin U 100 as the standard potency appears inevitable. Advantages of this single concentration of insulin include compatability with the metric system and reduction of errors resulting from the use of incorrectly calibrated syringes.

Comparison of insulin preparations*

Insulin	Onset (hours)	Peak (hours)	Duration (hours)
Rapid-acting			
Insulin injection U.S.P. (regular insulin)	½-1	3-5	5-8
Prompt insulin suspension U.S.P. (semilente insulin)	½-1	4-6	12-16
Intermediate-acting			
Insulin zinc suspension U.S.P. (lente insulin)	1-2	8-12	24-28
Isophane insulin suspension U.S.P. (N.P.H. insulin)	1-2	8-12	24-28
Long-acting			
Extended zinc insulin suspension U.S.P. (ultralente insulin)	5-8	16-18	36+
Protamine zinc suspension U.S.P. (protamine zinc)	1-1½	14-20	36+

*These figures are based on average figures of newly diagnosed, uncomplicated diabetic patients.

The only insulin preparation that can be given intravenously is regular (unmodified) insulin. All other insulin preparations are categorized based on the following three factors:

1. Onset: the time when insulin begins to act on the body
2. Peak: the time when the insulin exerts maximum action
3. Duration: the length of time the insulin remains in effect

MEASURING UNITS OF INSULIN

The simplest and most accurate way to measure insulin is with an insulin syringe. There are two 1-ml insulin syringes calibrated to insulin as follows on p. 129.

1. To the scale of U 40 in 1 ml and color-coded red (Fig. 6, *A*).
2. To the scale of U 100 in 1 ml and color-coded orange (Fig. 6, *B*).

Two types of syringes, 0.35 ml and 0.5 ml (Fig. 6, *C*), to be used for low doses of U 100 insulin are also available. It is important to measure U 40 insulin in a U 40 syringe, and U 100 insulin in a U 100 syringe. The standard insulin syringe is always a 1-ml syringe because the specified units (40 or 100) are contained in a 1-ml volume. Insulin in excess of 1 ml should never be administered.

An insulin syringe should consistently be used to measure insulin, but if it is not available a 2-ml (♏ 32) hypodermic syringe calibrated in fractions of ml and ♏ can also be used. The tuberculin syringe can also be used for measuring insulin. It is a 1-ml, double-scaled syringe, calibrated in fractions of a milliliter and in minims (Fig. 6, *D*). It is best to use the minim calibration in measuring insulin (1 ml = ♏ 16). Use the following formula:

$$\frac{D}{H} \times \text{quantity} = x \text{ (amount to be administered)}$$

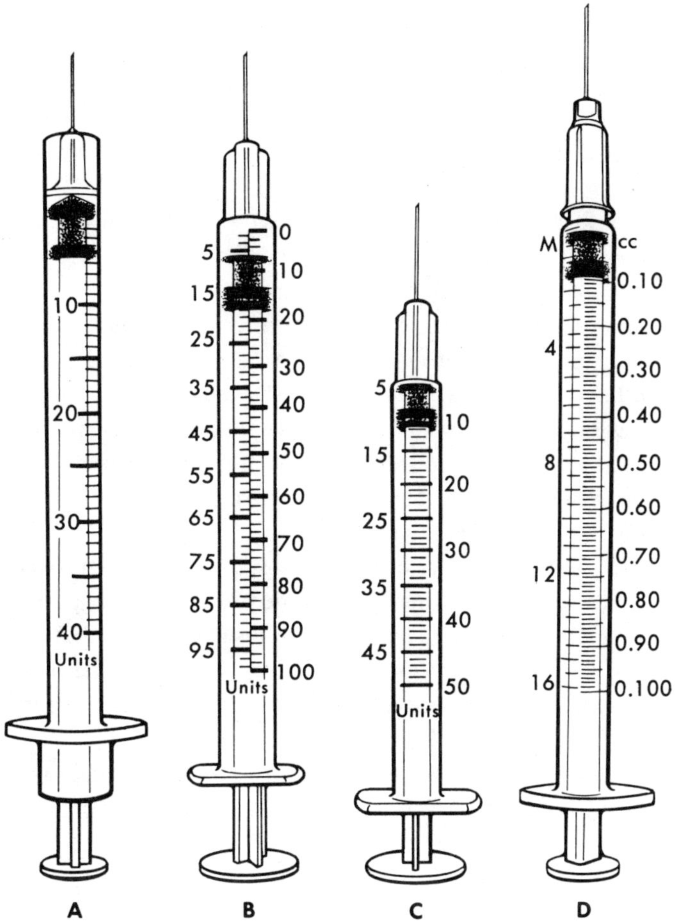

Fig. 6. Insulin syringes: **A,** U 40; **B,** U 100; **C,** U 100 low dose. **D,** Tuberculin syringe.

EXAMPLE: Measure 20 U of U 100 insulin, using a hypodermic syringe. D = 20 U; H = 100 U; quantity = 1 ml or 15 ♏.

$$\frac{20}{100} \times 15 = 3 \text{ ♏}$$

or

$$\frac{20 \text{ units}}{100 \text{ units}} = \frac{x \text{ minims}}{15 \text{ minims}}$$

$$100x = 300$$

$$x = 3 \text{ ♏}$$

The U 40 scale syringe has 40 calibrations, each calibration indicating 1 unit of U 40 insulin. To give an amount such as U 35 of U 40 insulin draw the solution up to the 35 calibration in the syringe.

The U 100 scale syringe has 50 calibrations, each calibration indicating 2 U of U 100 insulin. If U 50 of U 100 insulin is ordered, the solution is drawn up to the U 50 calibration.

The U 35 scale syringe (for use with U 100 insulin only) has 35 calibrations, each calibration indicating 1 unit of U 100 insulin. If U 15 of U 100 insulin is ordered, the solution is drawn up to the U 15 calibration.

Regular insulin may be added to NPH insulin to produce more rapid onset of action and intermediate duration of action. These mixtures should be used immediately after preparation because physical changes, which would result in unpredictable results, may occur on standing. Mixtures of regular and protamine zinc insulin may be prepared in advance, but because of an excess of protamine in protamine zinc insulin, predictable results are difficult to obtain. Mixtures of the lente preparation may be combined in any desired ratio and can be made in advance.

To obtain the dosage of two types of insulin to be given together, draw the regular insulin into the syringe first, then the modified insulin. Using proper technique will avoid contaminating the insulin preparations with insulin of the other type.

EXAMPLE: Give U 10 of regular insulin and U 30 of NPH insulin.

Use insulins of the same concentration. Use proper syringe to measure insulin in units or minims (after conversion from units to minims).

1. Observing sterile precautions, inject volume of air equal to dose (U 30 in example) into top of vial of modified (NPH) insulin. Withdraw needle.

2. Inject air and withdraw proper dose of regular insulin (U 10).

3. Invert vial of modified insulin and rotate several times. Withdraw dose (U 30) into syringe containing regular insulin.

LABORATORY PROBLEMS— Insulin

Name ______________________

Date ______________________

Equipment: U 40 and U 100 insulin syringes, 2-ml hypodermic syringes, tuberculin syringes and needles, and preparations of insulin* as indicated in the problems.

1. Use a U 40 insulin syringe and U 40 insulin to practice measuring the following:
   a. U 10
   b. U 40
   c. U 25
   d. U 8
2. Use a U 100 insulin syringe and U 100 insulin to practice measuring the following:
   a. U 10
   b. U 40
   c. U 25
   d. U 85
3. Using the tuberculin syringe measure:

   a. U 12 of U 40 insulin is ♏ ______________

   b. U 24 of U 40 insulin is ♏ ______________

   c. U 30 of U 100 insulin is ♏ ______________

   d. U 38 of U 100 insulin is ♏ ______________

4. Using a 2-ml hypodermic syringe, measure:

   a. U 10 of U 40 is ♏ ______________.

   b. U 40 of U 100 is ♏ ______________.

5. Using a 0.5-ml U 100 insulin syringe and U 100 insulin, measure the following:
   a. U 10
   b. U 14
   c. U 18
6. Mixtures of insulin. Using U 100 insulin and a U 100 syringe for practice,
   a. prepare regular insulin U 16 and NPH insulin U 30
   b. prepare regular insulin U 8 and Lente insulin U 30

*For practice, vials containing sterile water or saline can be substituted for insulin.

CALCULATING DOSES OF INTRAVENOUS FLUIDS AND ELECTROLYTES

Definite amounts of water and electrolytes are required by the body to maintain fluid balance and cellular functions. Almost any disease condition, surgical procedure or other injury, or malfunction of one or more body organs (such as the kidney) will produce a problem in fluid and electrolyte balance. The physician orders intravenous infusions containing water, dextrose for calories, and electrolytes such as sodium chloride to reestablish the body's internal balance. The nurse should be familiar with the terminology involved, be able to prepare the infusion, and add the ordered dose from concentrated electrolyte solutions.

The terms and calculations used in dosage determinations are explained in the following discussion to help the nurse better understand electrolyte therapy.

Electrolytes are chemical compounds in solution that dissociate or split to form ions. This process is called ionization. Examples of electrolytes are sodium chloride, potassium phosphate, and magnesium sulfate.

Ions are dissociated particles of an electrolyte. Some have a positive charge and others a negative charge. Ions with a positive charge (+) are called cations. Sodium (Na^+) is an example. Ions with a negative charge (−) are called anions. Chloride (Cl^-) is an example. Ions are often administered in intravenous solutions to correct deficiencies and to restore acid-base balance.

Milliequivalents

Doses of ions are calculated in milliequivalents (mEq). A milliequivalent is $1/1000$ of an equivalent weight. The equivalent weight of a compound is calculated by dividing the gram-molecular weight of the compound by the valence. (Valence is an expression of the combining capacity of an element as measured by the number of hydrogen atoms with which one atom of the element can combine.) For example:

$$\text{NaCl gram-molecular weight} = 58.5$$
$$(Na^+ = 23,\ Cl^- = 35.5) \text{ monovalent}$$
$$\text{Equivalent weight} = \frac{58.5}{1} = 58.5$$

$$Na_2SO_4 \text{ gram-molecular weight} = 142$$
$$(Na^+ \times 2 = 46,\ SO_4^= = 96) \text{ bivalent}$$
$$\text{Equivalent weight} = \frac{142}{2} = 71$$

Expressions in terms of equivalent weights are useful, since when gram units are converted to equivalents, the concentration of elements and compounds are expressed in terms of their combining weights. This reduces the units to a common expression, and equivalents of any and all substances involved can be added or compared mathematically. Total cations always equal total anions. They balance each other. This equality does not exist when electrolytes are expressed as milligrams per 100 ml. The expression milligrams percent (mg %) as commonly used is taken to mean milligrams per 100 ml.

To calculate equivalents use the formula

$$\text{equivalent} = \frac{\text{g}}{\text{equivalent weight}}$$

To calculate milliequivalents, use the formula

$$\text{mEq} = \frac{\text{mg}}{\text{equivalent weight}}$$

To determine the correct equivalent weight (EW) of a compound such as calcium chloride ($CaCl_2$), divide the molecular weight (MW) by the valence of either ion times the number of that ion represented by the formula of that compound.

EXAMPLE: $CaCl_2 = Ca^{++} + 2Cl^-$

Therefore the equivalent weight of $CaCl_2$ equals the molecular weight divided by (2) × (1).

$$\text{EW of } CaCl_2 = \frac{\text{MW}}{(2)\,(1)} = \frac{\text{MW}}{2}$$

EXAMPLE: A dose of 8 mEq of Mg^{++} is needed. A stock solution of 50% $MgSO_4$ (MW $MgSO_4$ = 246.47) is on hand. $MgSO_4 = Mg^{++} + SO_4^=$. 1 mEq $MgSO_4$ = 1 mEq Mg^{++} + 1 mEq $SO_4^=$, or 8 mEq $MgSO_4$ = 8 mEq Mg^{++}

$$\text{mEq} = \frac{\text{mg}}{\text{EW}}$$

$$8 = \frac{\text{mg}}{\text{EW}}$$

$$\text{EW} = \frac{246.47}{2}$$

$$8 = \frac{\text{mg}}{246.47/2} \quad \text{or} \quad 8 = \frac{2\,(\text{mg})}{246.47}$$

$$\text{mg} = 8 \times \frac{246.47}{2} = 985.88 \text{ mg or } 986 \text{ mg}$$

The 50% stock solution contains 50 g/100 ml or 1 g/2 ml or 1000 mg/2 ml.

$$\text{Then } \frac{1000 \text{ mg}}{2 \text{ ml}} = \frac{986 \text{ mg}}{x \text{ ml}}$$

$$x = \frac{2\,(986)}{1000} = 1.972 \text{ ml, or } 2 \text{ ml}$$

Two milliliters of a 50% stock solution of $MgSO_4$ would contain 8 mEq of Mg^{++}.

To convert milligrams per 100 ml (mg/100 ml) to milliequivalents per liter (mEq/l) the following formula has been developed:

$$\frac{\text{mg/100 ml} \times 10 \times \text{valence}}{\text{molecular weight}} = \frac{\text{mEq}}{\text{l}}$$

EXAMPLE: A chloride concentration is reported as 300 mg/100 ml. Its concentration in mEq/l is

$$\frac{300 \times 10 \times 1}{35.5} = 84.6 \text{ mEq/l}$$

35.5 = molecular weight of one equivalent of chloride

EXAMPLE: Normal saline contains 9 g of sodium chloride per liter (900 mg/100 ml)

$$\frac{900 \times 10 \times 1}{58.5} = 154 \text{ mEq/l of sodium or of chloride}$$

58.5 = molecular weight of sodium chloride

EXAMPLE: What is the concentration, in mg/ml, of a solution containing 3 mEq of potassium chloride (KCl) per milliliter?

Molecular weight of KCl = 74.5

Equivalent weight of KCl = 74.5

$$1 \text{ mEq of KCl} = \frac{74.5 \text{ g}}{1000} = 0.0745 \text{ g} = 74.5 \text{ mg}$$

$$3 \text{ mEq of KCl} = 74.5 \times 3 = 223.5 \text{ mg/ml}$$

EXAMPLE: A 10-ml ampule of potassium chloride contains 2.98 g of potassium chloride (MW KCl = 74.5). What is the concentration of the solution in terms of mEq/ml?

$$\text{mEq} = \frac{2980 \text{ mg}}{74.5} = 40 \text{ mEq/10 ml, or 4 mEq/ml}$$

EXAMPLE: How many grams of sodium chloride (MW NaCl = 58.5) should be used to prepare a solution containing 154 mEq/l?

$$154 = \frac{x}{58.5}$$

$$x = 9009 \text{ mg or } 9.009 \text{ g (9 g)}$$

It may be necessary for the nurse to calculate the volume of a concentrated ion solution to be added to an intravenous infusion.

EXAMPLE: Fifteen milliequivalents of potassium ion is to be added to a 5% dextrose solution for intravenous infusion. The K^+ is to be obtained from a vial of KCl containing 20 mEq of KCl in 20 ml of solution.

20 mEq:20 ml::15 mEq:x ml

x = 15 ml of the KCl solution to be added to provide 15 mEq of K^+

Millimoles

A mole is the molecular weight of a substance in grams. A millimole (mM) is 1/1000 of the molecular weight in grams.

Some groups of ions, such as phosphate, exist in both monovalent and divalent forms. Calculation of phosphate in milliequivalents requires knowledge of the relative proportions of monovalent ($H_2PO_4^-$) and divalent ($HPO_4^=$) phosphate. These proportions are determined by the acidity of the potassium phosphate preparation and the intravenous fluid with which it is mixed. As the acidity changes, so does the ratio between monovalent and divalent phosphates. Because this ratio is unknown, the desired dose of phosphate should be calculated in millimoles.

For example, the molecular weight of divalent phosphate is 95.98 g. Therefore one mole weighs 95.98 g, and one millimole would weigh 1/1000 of this or 95.98 mg.

EXAMPLE: How many mM of phosphate and how many mEq of potassium are present in a mixture containing 1.12 g of monobasic potassium phosphate (KH_2PO_4) and 1.18 g of dibasic potassium phosphate (K_2HPO_4)?

Given: Molecular weight for KH_2PO_4 = 136.09
Molecular weight for K_2HPO_4 = 174.18
One mEq potassium weighs 39.1 mg.

Because there is one phosphate radical/molecule in each case, the number of mM of phosphate will be numerically equal to the number of mM of the entire compound.

One mM of KH_2PO_4 weighs 136.09 mg, and one mM of K_2HPO_4 weighs 174.18 mg. Therefore,

$$\frac{1.12 \text{ g } KH_2PO_4}{136.09 \text{ mg/mM}} = 8.23 \text{ mM} \qquad \frac{1.18 \text{ g } K_2HPO_4}{174.18 \text{ mg/mM}} = 6.77 \text{ mM}$$

Adding 8.23 and 6.77 mM, we find there are 15 mM of phosphate present in this mixture.

To find out how many mEq of potassium are present, first determine the percent potassium by weight in each compound.

For KH_2PO_4: $\frac{39.1}{136.09} = 28.73\% \ K^+$

For K_2HPO_4: $\frac{78.2}{174.18} = 44.90\% \ K^+$

Now determine the weight of potassium in each compound.

For KH_2PO_4: 28.73% of 1.12 g = 321.8 mg K^+

For K_2HPO_4: 44.90% of 1.18 g = 529.8 mg K^+

The two compounds contribute a total of 851.6 mg potassium. Converting this value into mEq of potassium, we have:

$$\frac{851.6 \text{ mg } K^+}{39.1 \text{ mg } K^+/\text{mEq}} = 21.78 \text{ mEq } K^+$$

Note that the number of mM of phosphate (15 mM) is not the same as the mEq of potassium (22 mEq).

Milliosmoles

Electrolytes help in controlling body water volumes by establishing osmotic pressure. This pressure is proportional to the total number of particles in solution. The milliosmole (mOsm) is the unit used to measure osmotic activity. For nonelectrolytes such as dextrose, 1 millimole represents 1 milliosmole. For electrolytes the total number of particles in solution depends on the degree of dissociation. Assuming complete dissolution, 1 millimole of KCl represents 2 milliosmoles (K^+ and Cl^-) of total particles, and 1 millimole of $CaCl_2$ represents 3 milliosmoles (Ca^+ and 2 Cl^-) of total particles.

EXAMPLE: A solution contains 10% of anhydrous dextrose in water for injection. How many milliosmoles per liter are represented by this concentration?

Molecular weight of dextrose = 180

1 millimole (180 mg) = 1 milliosmole

10% solution contains 100 g or 100,000 mg/l

100,000 mg ÷ 180 = 555.5 mOsm/l

EXAMPLE: How many milliosmoles are represented in a liter of 0.9% sodium chloride solution?

Molecular weight of NaCl = 58.5

1 millimole (58.5 mg) = 2 milliosmoles

0.009 × 1000 = 9 g or 9000 mg NaCl/l

$$x = \frac{2 \times 9000}{58.5}$$

$$x = 307.7 \text{ mOsm}$$

FLOW RATES FOR INTRAVENOUS SOLUTIONS

The rate of flow at which an intravenous infusion is administered is ordered by the physician. However, the nurse is often given the responsibility of regulating and maintaining this rate of flow. Intravenous sets are equipped with a drip chamber, which is a short tube inserted into the bottle cap and connected to the tubing and needle assembly. The drip chamber contains a small-diameter tube through which drops form as the infusion flows. The flow rate is adjusted by means of a clamp placed on the tubing. The dropper in the drip chamber is calibrated, and each set is labeled with this calibration. The drops per milliliter calibration of the solution administration set is sometimes referred to as the "Standard Drop Factor." Because intravenous solutions are of the same approximate viscosity, the same calibration can be used for the administration of various solutions.

Flow rates for intravenous infusions are determined by using the following formula:

$$\frac{\text{drops/ml of given set}}{\text{60 (minutes in hour)}} \times \text{total hourly volume} = \text{drops/min}$$

EXAMPLE: The physician orders 200 ml to be infused in 1 hour. The administration set is calibrated to deliver 15 drops/ml.

$$\frac{15}{60} \times 200 = 50 \text{ drops/min}$$

EXAMPLE: The physician orders 5% dextrose in 0.2% saline 1000 ml with 30 mEq KCl to be infused over 8 hours. What is the correct infusion rate in milliliters per hour and in drops per minute? The Standard Drop Factor of the administration set is 10.

The infusion rate in milliliters per hour is determined by dividing the total volume to be infused by the total time for infusion:

$$\frac{1000 \text{ ml}}{8 \text{ hr}} = 125 \text{ ml/hr}$$

The infusion rate in ml/min is determined by dividing the rate in ml/hr by 60 (minutes per hour).

$$\frac{125 \text{ ml/hr}}{60 \text{ min/hr}} = 2.1 \text{ ml/min}$$

The infusion rate in drops per minute is determined by multiplying the rate in milliliters per minute by the Standard Drop Factor (the drops per milliliter measured by the solution administration set used).

$$2.1 \text{ ml/min} \times 10 = 21 \text{ drops/min}$$

The infusion rate may be altered during the course of administration because of factors such as position changes of the patient. The nurse must then recalculate the flow rate to infuse the intravenous fluid in the ordered amount of time.

The following formula is used to recalculate the rate of an already infusing intravenous solution.

$$\frac{\begin{array}{c}\text{total amount of solution} \\ \text{in ml left to be infused}\end{array} \times \text{standard drop factor}}{\text{number of hours remaining} \times 60 \text{ minutes}} = \text{drops/minute}$$

EXAMPLE: There are 400 ml left in an infusing bottle of 1000 ml 5% dextrose in water. The fluid must be infused over the next 3 hours. What should the new rate be using equipment with a Standard Drop Factor of 10?

$$\frac{400 \text{ ml} \times 10}{3 \times 60} = \frac{4000}{180} = 22 \text{ drops/minute}$$

EQUIPMENT FOR MONITORING FLOW RATES

Major fluctuations in flow rate occur with gravity-fed infusion of intravenous fluids under clinical conditions. As a result, mechanical infusion pumps have been developed to rectify this problem and assure accurate fluid delivery. Technologic developments in electronic microcircuitry have enabled the health products industry to market volumetric infusion pumps that are versatile, reliable, and moderately priced. The pumps are similar in design and consist of a pump chamber that is incorporated into a disposable plastic administration set. A piston from the infusion pump connects to the administration set pump chamber and supplies the mechanical energy to pump the intravenous solution. A computer chip within the infusion pump oversees the cycle times and by this means regulates the infusion rate and volume of solution to be administered.

Volumetric infusion pumps have been useful for the infusion of potent medications where constancy in the flow rate is mandatory to prevent serious complications. The flow rate can be mechanically set to deliver from 1 to 999 ml/hr with 1-ml increments. Monitoring of the infusion is provided by audible and visual alarm mechanisms.

DOSAGE OF HYPERALIMENTATION THERAPY

Hyperalimentation, or total parenteral nutrition (TPN), is a method of providing the complete nutritional needs of a patient by the intravenous route (generally the subclavian vein). Patients who are unable to supply their nutritional needs adequately by the oral route and who will not be expected to resume normal eating patterns within a few days are candidates for TPN. This therapy is primarily used to help patients heal more rapidly and efficiently after surgical procedures and to survive prolonged illness such as cancer.

Designing a parenteral nutrition formula that meets the patient's daily requirements is a complex task. The patient's body surface area can be used to determine daily fluid requirements. The guideline is 1500 ml/m^2/day. Therefore, a patient with a surface area of 1.7 m^2 would need 2550 ml/day. Additional fluid volume is replaced if the patient has a fever (300 to 700 ml/day for each degree over normal) or is experiencing excessive fluid losses. Dextrose is most frequently used as a calorie source. It supplies 3.4 Kcal/g. Most people require between 2000 and 3000 Kcal/day. The stress of illness increases the caloric requirements. Methods to calculate the number of calories required to meet daily energy expenditure are available for individual patient needs. Intravenous fat in the form of linoleic acid is also used to provide calories and to prevent essential fatty acid deficiencies. It supplies 9.1 Kcal/g. Protein or a nitrogen source is supplied by crystalline amino acid solutions; 1 g of nitrogen equals 6.25 g of protein. Normal requirements are 70 g of protein or 11 g of nitrogen per day. Increases in metabolic demands require increases in nitrogen requirements.

If an 8.5% crystalline amino acid solution containing 6.25 g of nitrogen and a 50% dextrose solution is used, a final mixture containing 4.25% amino acids and 25% dextrose in 1 liter can be prepared. This contains:

1. 1000 ml of water
2. 250 g dextrose × 3.4 Kcal/g = 850 Kcal
3. 6.25 g of nitrogen

Between 2.5 and 3 liters of this solution will provide the normal fluid, caloric, and nitrogen requirements.

Electrolytes, vitamins, and trace elements are added to maintain normal values or correct abnormalities.

A parenteral nutrition formula (per liter) may be ordered as follows:

Bottle No. 1 Sodium chloride 60 mEq
Potassium phosphate 9 mM
Potassium acetate 20 mEq
Calcium gluconate 5 mEq
Multivitamin conc. 5 ml
Dextrose 25%
Crystalline amino acids 4.25%

Bottle No. 2 Sodium chloride 60 mEq
Potassium phosphate 9 mM
Potassium acetate 20 mEq
Magnesium sulfate 8 mEq
Folic acid 1 mg
Dextrose 25%
Crystalline amino acids 4.25%

Bottle No. 3 Sodium chloride 60 mEq
Potassium phosphate 9 mM
Potassium acetate 20 mEq
Dextrose 25%
Crystalline amino acids 4.25%

ADULT DOSAGE BASED ON SURFACE AREA METHOD

The surface area method of calculating drug dosage is an accurate means of determining dosage for parenteral administration, particularly in situations in which the dose must be very carefully calibrated. This method may also be used for determining dosages for oral administration. This method requires finding the body surface area in square meters. Nomograms are available and can be used to determine the body surface area when the height and weight are known. The use of the West nomogram is described in Chapter 13.

PROBLEMS

Name ____________________

Date ____________________

PARENTERAL DOSAGE

Dosage of drugs from stock on hand in vials or ampules. Round off fraction of minims to the nearest measurable dose.

1. Prostigmin from a 1:1000 solution. Prepare (a) 0.3 mg; (b) 1 mg.

   a. ______________; b. ______________

2. Atropine sulfate from a vial in which there are 0.6 mg/ml. Prepare (a) 1.2 mg; (b) 0.8 mg.

   a. ______________; b. ______________

3. Robinul from a 20-ml vial in which there are 0.2 mg/ml. Prepare (a) gr $\frac{1}{250}$; (b) gr $\frac{1}{200}$.

   a. ______________; b. ______________

4. Synkayvite ampules 1 ml containing 2.5 mg, 5 mg, and 10 mg. Which ampule would you use to give (a) 2 mg; (b) 8 mg. How much?

   a. ______________; b. ______________

5. Levo-Dromoran from a vial labeled 10 ml = 20 mg. Give (a) 3 mg; (b) 2.5 mg.

a. ________; b. ________

6. Methadone hydrochloride from a 10-ml vial in which there are 10 mg in 1 ml. Prepare (a) 15 mg; (b) 5 mg.

a. ________; b. ________

7. Codeine sulfate from vial labeled 60 mg in 1 ml. Prepare (a) gr $\frac{3}{4}$; (b) gr $\frac{1}{2}$.

a. ________; b. ________

8. Morphine sulfate from vial labeled gr v in 20 ml. Prepare (a) gr $\frac{1}{4}$; (b) gr $\frac{1}{6}$; (c) gr $\frac{1}{8}$.

a. ________; b. ________; c. ________

PROBLEMS

Name ______________________

Date ______________________

PARENTERAL DOSAGE—cont'd

9. Meperidine hydrochloride from ampule labeled 100 mg in 2 ml. Prepare (a) gr i; (b) gr iss.

a. ____________; b. ____________

10. Dilaudid from vial labeled 40 mg in 20 ml. Prepare (a) 2.5 mg; (b) 3 mg.

a. ____________; b. ____________

11. Meperidine hydrochloride labeled 1000 mg in 20-ml vial. Prepare (a) 100 mg; (b) 75 mg.

a. ____________; b. ____________

12. Fluorouracil ampules labeled 500 mg/10 ml. Prepare 750 mg.

____

13. Mannitol from a 25% solution. Prepare 50 g.

____

14. Thorazine from vial labeled 25 mg in 1 ml. Prepare 15 mg.

____

15. Phenergan from a vial labeled 25 mg in 1 ml. Prepare gr $\frac{3}{4}$.

____

16. Cortisone from a 20-ml vial labeled 500 mg. Prepare (a) 75 mg; (b) 25 mg.

a. ____________; b. ____________

17. Lanoxin from an ampule labeled 0.25 mg in 1 ml. Prepare 0.15 mg.

____

PROBLEMS

Name ______________________

Date ______________________

PARENTERAL DOSAGE—cont'd

18. Prostigmin from a 1:2000 solution. Prepare 0.25 mg (gr $^1/_{250}$).

____

19. Ascorbic acid (vitamin C) from ampule labeled 500 mg in 2 ml. Prepare 0.25 g.

____

20. Vitamin K from ampule labeled 2 mg in 1 ml. Prepare gr $^1/_{15}$.

____

21. Cyanocobalamin from vial labeled 1000 μg in 10 ml. Prepare 250 μg.

____

22. Vitamin B_{12} ampule labeled 100 μg in 1 ml. Prepare 60 μg.

____

23. Tubocurarine from a 10-ml vial labeled 3 mg in 1 ml. Prepare 5 mg.

____

24. Heparin sodium from a 5-ml vial labeled 10,000 U in 1 ml. Prepare (a) 15,000 U; (b) 40,000 U.

a. ____________; b. ____________

25. Betalin-12 from a 5-ml vial labeled 1000 μg in 1 ml. Prepare 750 μg.

____

26. Erythromycin gluceptate from a bottle labeled 1000 mg in 20 ml. Prepare 0.25 g for I.V.

____

27. A vial of penicillin solution contains the following units.

a. 500,000 U/ml. Give 600,000 U ____________

b. 400,000 U/ml. Give 600,000 U ____________

c. 200,000 U/ml. Give 150,000 U ____________

d. 100,000 U/ml. Give 900,000 U ____________

PROBLEMS

Name ______________________

Date ______________________

PARENTERAL DOSAGE—cont'd

28. Stock vials of penicillin contain
    a. 5,000,000 U. Dilute to
        (1) 300,000 U in 1 ml. ______________
        (2) 500,000 U in 1 ml. ______________
    b. 1,000,000 U. Dilute to
        (1) 50,000 U in 1 ml. ______________
        (2) 250,000 U in 1 ml. ______________

29. How many milliliters are needed to give 25 mg of meperidine from a 30-ml vial labeled 50 mg/ml?

____

30. How many milliliters are needed to give gr $^3/_4$ of phenobarbital from a 2-ml ampule containing gr ii?

____

31. On hand is a 10-ml vial of Dilaudid labeled 2 mg/ml. How many milliliters are needed to give a dose of gr $^1/_{20}$?

____

32. A stock solution of morphine sulfate is available containing gr 5 in 20 ml. How much is needed to give gr $\frac{1}{4}$?

____

33. How many milliliters are needed to prepare gr $7\frac{1}{2}$ of magnesium sulfate from a 2-ml ampule labeled 1 g?

____

34. How many milliliters are needed to give a 40-mg dose of Lasix from an ampule containing 100 mg/10 ml?

____

35. On hand is a 20-ml ampule of magnesium sulfate containing 2 g. How many milliliters are needed to give 750 mg?

____

36. A vial of Solu-Medrol contains 40 mg/ml. How much is needed to give 30 mg?

____

37. A stock solution is available containing 100 U in 10 ml. How much is needed to give 20 U?

____

PROBLEMS

Name ______________________

Date ______________________

PARENTERAL DOSAGE—cont'd

38. How many milliliters of sodium heparin are needed to give 1500 units from a stock solution containing 50,000 units in 5 ml?

 ____

39. A vial of Valium contains 5 mg/ml. How much is needed to give 2 mg?

 ____

40. How many milliliters are needed to give a 50-mg dose of Talwin from a vial labeled 300 mg/10 ml?

 ____

Measuring mEq, mM, and mOsm

Solve the following problems:

1. How many milliliters of a solution containing 40 mEq of KCl per 12.5 ml of solution would you need to prepare the following doses?

   a. 20 mEq potassium ion ____________

   b. 30 mEq potassium ion ____________

   c. 15 mEq potassium ion ____________

   d. 10 mEq potassium ion ____________

   e. 40 mEq potassium ion ____________

2. How many milliliters of a solution containing 10 mEq of KCl per 10 ml of solution would you need to prepare the following doses?

a. 8 mEq chloride ion ____________

b. 20 mEq chloride ion ____________

c. 12 mEq chloride ion ____________

d. 15 mEq chloride ion ____________

e. 35 mEq chloride ion ____________

3. How many milliliters of a solution containing 4 mEq of Mg^{++} per milliliter would you need to prepare the following doses of magnesium ion?

a. 8 mEq magnesium ion ____________

b. 16 mEq magnesium ion ____________

c. 6 mEq magnesium ion ____________

d. 12 mEq magnesium ion ____________

e. 20 mEq magnesium ion ____________

4. How many milliliters of a potassium phosphate solution containing 30 mEq K^{+}/10 ml would you need to prepare the following doses?

a. 20 mEq potassium ion ____________

b. 15 mEq potassium ion ____________

c. 10 mEq potassium ion ____________

d. 40 mEq potassium ion ____________

e. 60 mEq potassium ion ____________

5. How many milliliters of a sodium chloride solution containing 855 mEq of sodium per liter would you need to prepare the following doses?

a. 30 mEq sodium ion ____________

b. 40 mEq sodium ion ____________

c. 25 mEq sodium ion ____________

d. 12 mEq sodium ion ____________

e. 10 mEq sodium ion ____________

PROBLEMS

Name ______________________

Date ______________________

PARENTERAL DOSAGE—cont'd

6. How many milliliters of potassium phosphate solution containing 3 mM per milliliter would you need to prepare 9 mM of phosphate?

   ____

7. How many milliliters of sodium acetate solution containing 2 mEq/ml would you need to prepare 30 mEq of sodium?

   ____

8. A 250-ml vial contains a 2 mEq/ml of potassium chloride. How many milliliters of this solution would you need to prepare 16 mEq of chloride?

   ____

9. A 15-ml vial contains 45 mM of sodium phosphate. How many milliliters are needed to prepare 3 mM of phosphate?

   ____

10. A 30-ml vial contains 60 mEq of potassium chloride. How many milliliters are needed to prepare 45 mEq of potassium?

    ____

11. How many mEq of Ca^{++} are present in 10 ml of a 10% calcium gluconate (MW = 430.38) solution?

____

12. How many grams of sodium bicarbonate ($NaHCO_3$)(MW = 84) should be used in preparing 1 liter of solution containing 44.6 mEq/50 ml?

____

13. A patient received 1 liter of D5 ½ NS (5% dextrose with 0.45% NaCl) during intravenous fluid replacement therapy. How many mEq of Na^+ did he receive? (MW NaCl = 58.5)

____

14. How many milliosmoles are there in 100 ml of 10% calcium chloride solution ($CaCl_2 \cdot 2\ H_2O$)? (MW Ca = 40, Cl = 35.5, H = 1, O = 16)

____

15. How many milliosmoles of dextrose (MW 180) are present in 500 ml of 50% dextrose solution?

____

PROBLEMS

Name ______________________

Date ______________________

PARENTERAL DOSAGE—cont'd

Flow rate

Solve the following problems using a solution administration set with a Standard Drop Factor of 10:

1. 500 ml of intravenous fluid is to be infused in 3 hours. What is the infusion rate in drops per minute?

   ____

2. A total of 3000 ml of 5% Dextrose in 0.45% saline is to be infused over the next 24 hours. What is the infusion rate in drops per minute?

   ____

3. Give 50 ml of an antibiotic solution intravenously in the next 30 minutes. What should the infusion rate be in drops per minute?

   ____

4. 5% Dextrose in water 1000 ml is to be infused over the next 12 hours. (a) What is the infusion rate in ml/hr; (b) in drops/min? (c) After 4 hours, 500 ml are left. Recalculate the flow rate.

   a. ______________; b. ______________; c. ______________

5. Aminophyllin 0.5 g in 250 ml sterile distilled water is ordered I.V. to be given in 1 hour. How fast should the solution run?

   ____

Solve the following problems using a solution administration set with a Standard Drop Factor of 15:

6. Give 100 ml of tobramycin in 5% dextrose in water in the next 60 minutes. What should the infusion rate be in drops per minute?

____

7. Isuprel 1 mg is added to 500 ml of 5% dextrose in water. The infusion rate is 5 μg/min. What should the infusion rate be in drops per minute?

____

8. Levophed 4 ml has been added to 1000 ml of 5% dextrose in water. Each milliliter of this dilution contains 4 μg of Levophed base. The infusion rate is 2 μg/min. What should the infusion rate be in drops per minute?

____

9. Lidocaine is administered at the rate of 50 μg/kg/min. One gram of lidocaine has been added to 1 liter of 5% dextrose in water. What should the infusion rate be in drops per minute for an adult weighing 154 pounds?

____

10. There are 700 ml left in an infusing bottle of 1000 ml 5% dextrose in water. The fluid must be infused over the next 4 hours. What should the new infusion rate be?

____

CHAPTER 13

Pediatric Dosage

OBJECTIVES

At the completion of this chapter, the student will:

- calculate pediatric dosage using Clark's Rule, Young's Rule, and Fried's Rule
- calculate pediatric dosage using surface area method

Children are unique individuals who require specialized approaches to care. Part of their care program includes careful calculation of medication doses. These calculations are frequently based on a fraction of the adult dose, according to the child's age and/or body weight. Clark's Rule, Young's Rule, and Fried's Rule use this method of dosage calculation. The surface area method for determining children's dosages uses the surface area of the child and is a more reliable method of dosage calculation.

Physicians prescribe the drug dosages for children, but nurses should be able to determine dosages and recognize usual dosages for commonly administered drugs. Correct dosage for infants and children is critical.

CLARK'S RULE

Clark's Rule uses the weight of the child to determine the dose.

FORMULA: $\text{child's dose} = \dfrac{\text{weight in pounds}}{150 \text{ (average weight of adults)}} \times \text{adult dose}$

Problem

The adult dose of phenobarbital is gr 1 (60 mg). What is the dose for a child weighing 75 pounds? For an infant weighing 15 pounds? Using the preceding formula:

1. $\dfrac{75}{150} \times 60 = x$

$$x = \frac{75}{150} \times 60 = \frac{3}{\cancel{6}} \times \overset{10}{\cancel{60}} = 30$$

$x = 30$ mg for a child weighing 75 lb

2. $\frac{15}{150} \times 60 = x$

$$x = \frac{1}{\cancel{10}} \times \overset{6}{\cancel{60}} = 6$$

$x = 6$ mg for an infant weighing 15 lb

FRIED'S RULE

Fried's Rule is used for an infant 2 years of age or under.

FORMULA: $\text{child's dose} = \frac{\text{age in months}}{150 \text{ (average adult weight)}} \times \text{adult dose}$

Problem

The physician orders a medication for an infant 7 months of age. The adult dose is 15 ml, or ½ fl ℥. What is the infant dose?

1. $\frac{7}{\underset{10}{\cancel{150}}} \times \cancel{15} = \frac{7}{10}$ or 0.7 ml for an infant 7 months of age

2. ½ fl ℥ = ♏ 225

$\frac{7}{\underset{2}{\cancel{150}}} \times \overset{3}{\cancel{225}} = \frac{21}{2}$ or ♏ 10.5 for an infant 7 months of age

YOUNG'S RULE

Young's Rule is used when the child is more than 1 year of age and not over 12 years of age.

FORMULA: $\text{child's dose} = \frac{\text{age}}{\text{age in years} + 12} \times \text{adult dose}$

Problem

The adult dose of Seconal is 100 mg. What is the dose for a child 10 years of age?

$$\frac{10}{10 + 12} \times 100 = \frac{1000}{22} = \frac{500}{11} \text{ or 45 mg}$$

SURFACE AREA METHOD

The surface area method requires finding the surface area in square meters. This is the most accurate method of calculating a child's dosage and can be used for all children except newborn babies. Adult dosages of drugs can also be determined by the surface area method. Simple slide rules or nomograms, also available in charts, can be used in

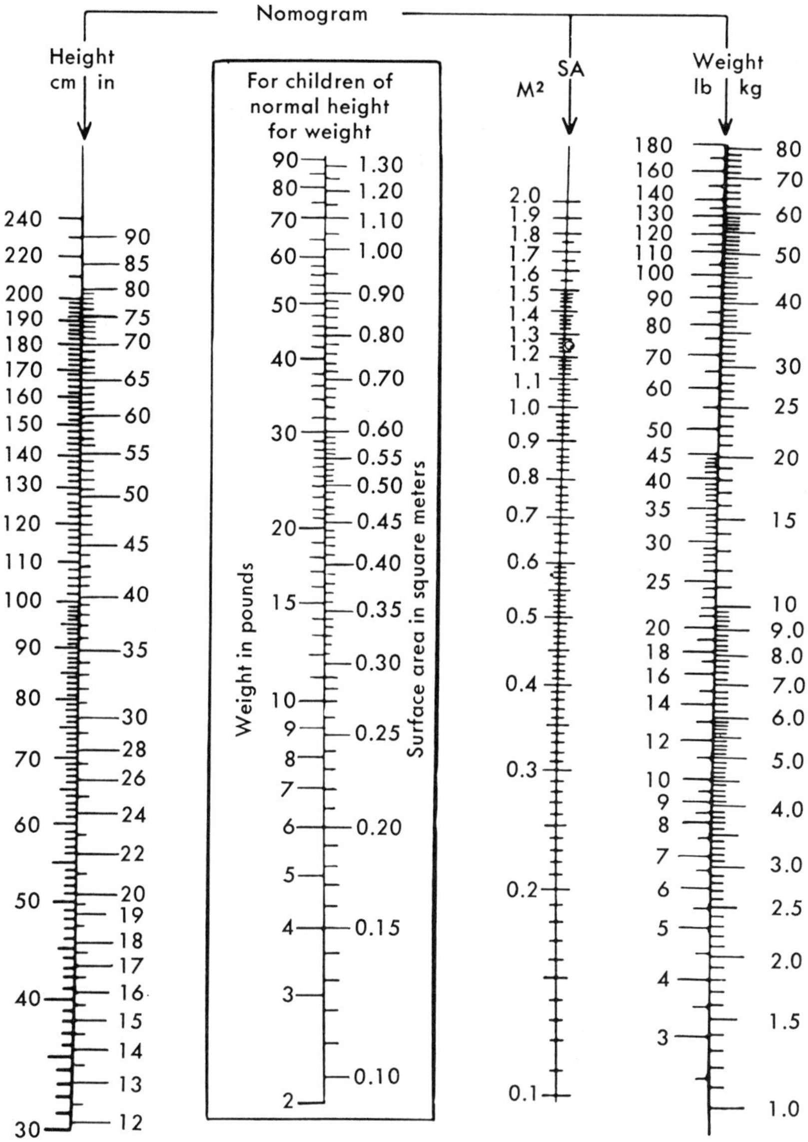

Fig. 7. West nomogram (for estimation of surface areas). The surface area is indicated where a straight line connecting the height and weight intersects the surface areas (SA) column or, if the patient is roughly of normal proportion, from the weight alone (enclosed area). (Nomogram modified from data of E. Boyd by C. D. West; from Shirkey, H. C.: Drug therapy. In Vaughn, V. C., III, and McKay, R. J., editors: Nelson's textbook of pediatrics, ed. 10, Philadelphia, 1975, W. B. Saunders Co.)

obtaining body surface area. The West nomogram (Fig. 7) has the height, weight, and surface area, in addition to an enclosed area for rapid conversion to surface area from weight alone.

$$\text{FORMULA: child's dose} = \frac{\text{child's body surface in m}^2}{1.7 \text{ (adult body surface in m}^2)} \times \text{adult dose}$$

The average surface area of 1.7 square meters has been accepted for adults.

Problem

A child's height is 100 cm and his weight is 20 kg. According to the nomogram, his body surface area (B.S.A.) is 0.76 m^2. The average adult dose of a drug is 100 mg. What is the dose for this child?

$$\frac{0.76}{1.7} \times 100 = 44.8 \text{ mg}$$

PROBLEMS

Name ______________________

Date ______________________

PEDIATRIC DOSAGE

Solve the following problems:

1. If the adult dose of a drug is 0.6 g to 2 g (gr x to xxx):
   a. Find the dose for a child weighing 37.5 pounds using the minimum dosage.

   ____

   b. Repeat, using the maximum dosage.

   ____

   c. The solution is prepared so that 4 ml is equivalent to 0.3 g (gr v). How much of the solution will be required to give the first dose?

   ____

   d. The second dose?

   ____

2. The adult dosage of epinephrine chloride (Adrenalin) is 0.2 mg to 1 mg given subcutaneously or intramuscularly.
   a. Find the dose for a child weighing 80 pounds, using the minimum dosage.

   ____

   b. Repeat, using the maximum dosage.

   ____

3. The adult dosage of cortisone is 100 mg/day. What is the dosage for a child weighing 75 pounds?

____

4. The adult dosage of procaine penicillin is 600,000 U to 1,200,000 U daily.
   a. Using the maximum dosage, calculate the dose for a child weighing 60 pounds.

   ____

   b. The solution is prepared so that each milliliter supplies 300,000 U. What fraction of a milliliter do you give this child?

   ____

   c. How many minims is this?

   ____

5. Recommended dosage of erythromycin is 300 to 800 mg a day. Using the minimum dosage, calculate (a) the total daily dosage and (b) the amount of medication per dose for an infant 10 months of age if the drug is given every 6 hours.

a. ______________; b. ______________

PROBLEMS

Name ____________________

Date ____________________

PEDIATRIC DOSAGE—cont'd

6. The adult dose of chloral hydrate is 0.5 g (gr viiss).
   a. What is the dose for a 3-year-old child?

   ____

   b. How can you give this amount from a solution in which 4 ml = 0.3 g (fl ʒ i = gr v)?

   ____

7. A child weighs 10 pounds. How many grains of aspirin would be ordered if the dosage is given using Clark's Rule? (Usual adult dose is gr x.)

   ____

8. The adult dose of a drug is 0.6 ml (♏ 10). What is the dose for a child weighing 95 pounds?

   ____

9. The adult dose of Luminal is 0.016 to 0.3 g (gr ¼ to v).
   a. What is the dose for a 5-year-old child using minimum dose?

   ____

   b. What is the dose using maximum dose?

   ____

10. The total daily dose of Dilantin is 100 mg to 300 mg.
    a. What is the dose for a child weighing 35.6 pounds using the minimum dose?

    ____

    b. What is the dose using the maximum dose?

    ____

11. The adult dose of codeine sulfate is 30 mg (gr ss). What is the dose for a 2-year-old child?

    ____

PROBLEMS

Name ______________________

Date ______________________

PEDIATRIC DOSAGE—cont'd

12. The average dose of Lomotil is 2 teaspoonfuls (10 ml) for adults. Each 5 ml contains 2.5 mg diphenoxylate and 0.025 mg atropine. What is the dose for a child whose weight is 45 pounds?

    ____

13. An average adult dose of ampicillin is 250 mg. What is the dose for a child whose weight is 30 pounds?

    ____

14. The body surface area of a child weighing 30 pounds is 0.6 m^2. The average adult dose of a drug is 500 mg to 1000 mg.
    a. What is the dose for this child using the maximum dose?

    ____

    b. What is the dose for this child using the minimum dose?

    ____

15. The average adult dose of a drug is 1 g. What is the dose for a 4-year-old child?

    ____

16. The adult dose of a drug is 75 mg to 100 mg.
    a. What is the dose for a 6-month-old child using the maximum dose?

    ____

    b. What is the dose for a 6-month-old child using the minimum dose?

    ____

17. According to the nomogram, the body surface area is 0.59 for a child whose height is 80 cm and whose weight is 15 kg. The average adult dose of a drug is 1 mg. What is the dose for this child?

    ____

18. The body surface area of a child is 0.9. The average adult dose of a drug is 60 mg. What is the dose for this child?

    ____

PROBLEMS

Name ____________________

Date ____________________

PEDIATRIC DOSAGE—cont'd

19. The average adult dose of a drug is 8 to 15 mg. What is the dose for a child whose body surface area is 1.0?
    a. What is maximum dose?

    ____

    b. What is minimum dose?

    ____

20. The average adult dose of a drug is 250 mg. What is the dose for a 20-pound child whose body surface area is 0.34?

    ____

21. Mintezol is ordered for a 33-pound child. The dose is 25 mg/kg body weight to be given twice a day for 1 day and the regimen repeated in 7 days. What is the total amount of Mintezol that will be administered to the child?

    ____

22. Kanamycin 7.5 mg/kg body weight is ordered for a 11-pound child to be given I.M. How many milliliters are needed from a vial containing 75 mg/2 ml?

____

23. The usual dose of vincristine for children is 2 mg/m^2. What is the dose for a child with a body surface area of 0.7 m^2?

____

24. Chlorambucil has been ordered for a 4-year-old child weighing 44 pounds. The dose is 0.2 mg/kg body weight daily for 21 days. How many 2-mg chlorambucil tablets are needed for the treatment?

____

25. Cytoxan has been ordered for a 7-year-old child weighing 55 pounds. The dose is 4 mg/kg body weight I.V. twice weekly. How much Cytoxan is needed for each dose?

____

APPENDIXES

- Drug Standards and Legal Regulations
- Common Arithmetic Terms
- Tables of Abbreviations and Equivalents
- Summary of Pediatric Dosage Rules
- Survey Test
- Comprehensive Examination for Review
- Answers to Problems

APPENDIX A

Drug Standards and Legal Regulations

UNITED STATES DRUG LEGISLATION

Recognition of the importance of establishing standards of quality and purity of drugs occurred in this century. The first federal legislation regulating the quality of drugs was the **Pure Food and Drug Act** of 1906. This law was passed to prevent the marketing of adulterated drugs and to eliminate labeling that made false and misleading claims. This Act also recognized two compendia as official books of drug standards. These books, *The United States Pharmacopeia* (U.S.P.) and the *National Formulary* (N.F.), define a drug's source, physical and chemical properties, and establish tests to determine its purity and identity. The U.S.P. and the N.F. provide the official names of drugs, information about the average dosage, methods of administration, and storage conditions. They are published every 5 years. The Board of Trustees of the U.S.P. and the N.F. determined that U.S.P. XX and N.F. XV be published in a single volume in 1980. The publication is devoted to standards and specifications of strength, quality, purity, packaging, and labeling for drugs and related articles. A separate volume entitled *U.S.P. Dispensing Information* contains dose and dispensing information and a section on drug advice for patients.

It is necessary to standardize drugs to ensure accurate dosage and reliability of effect. The technique by which the strength or potency of a drug is measured is known as **assay.** Drugs may be assayed by (1) chemical analysis to determine the ingredients present and their strength, and (2) biologic methods utilizing laboratory animals.

The **Federal Food, Drug, and Cosmetic Act** was passed in 1938 because of public pressure to ensure the safety of drug products. The law provides measures to prevent misbranding, adulterating, and incorporating harmful substances into foods, drugs, and cosmetics. It provides for mandatory testing of drugs in animals for possible toxicity prior to marketing. Enforcement of this Act is the responsibility of the Food and Drug Administration (F.D.A.) of the Department of Health and Human Services. Safety studies of drugs are reviewed by the F.D.A. before a new drug is allowed to be marketed.

The 1938 Act was amended in 1952 by the **Durham-Humphrey Amendment.** This prohibited the sale of drugs considered unsafe for self-medication without a prescription and restricted the refilling of prescriptions.

The **Kefauver-Harris Amendment** in 1962 empowered the F.D.A. to regulate procedures for testing drugs in humans. The major objectives were to ensure effectiveness as well as safety of drugs and to improve communication between manufacturers, prescribers, pharmacists, and consumers concerning effectiveness, side effects, and contraindications.

Proof of effectiveness is also required for drugs marketed before passage of the Kefauver-Harris Amendment. Thousands of older drugs have been or are in the process of being reevaluated. Drugs rated as "less than effective" in these studies are in the process of being removed from the market. Other drugs have been given a "probably" or "possibly" effective rating until further studies can establish definite effectiveness.

The first federal act to prevent drug addiction and regulate the importation, manufacture, sale, and use of opium and cocaine and all their compounds and derivatives was the **Harrison Narcotic Act** of 1914. Later regulations included marijuana and its derivatives and other drugs with habit-forming and addictive properties. Continuing abuse of drugs led to the passage of the **Narcotic Control Act** of 1956, which increased penalties for violation of the Harrison law and made possession of heroin unlawful. The **Drug Abuse Control Amendments** of 1965 increased regulations over central nervous system depressants such as barbiturates and stimulants such as amphetamines.

The Comprehensive Drug Abuse Prevention and Control Act of 1970 has replaced all former federal legislation regulating narcotics and dangerous drugs with abuse potential including the 1914, 1956, and 1965 regulations. A section of this 1970 Act known as the **Controlled Substances Act** schedules or classifies drugs according to medical usefulness and potential for abuse. Five schedules of controlled substances have been established.

Schedule I. Drugs with high-abuse potential that currently do not have accepted medical use, for example, heroin, marijuana, LSD (lysergic acid diethylamide).

Schedule II. Drugs that have medical use and a high-abuse potential, for example, morphine, amphetamine, secobarbital.

Schedule III. Drugs that have medical use and less potential for abuse than those in Schedule II, for example, codeine combined with a nonscheduled drug.

Schedule IV. Certain tranquilizers such as diazepam and sedatives such as chloral hydrate.

Schedule V. Over-the-counter drugs, for example, terpin hydrate with codeine, Robitussin A.C.

Under the guidelines of the 1970 Act, programs are developed and funded for drug education, treatment and rehabilitation for drug-dependent persons, and investigation of various aspects of the use of marijuana.

State laws also regulate the use of drugs. A state law may be more stringent but never more lenient than the federal law.

A nurse may possess narcotics or controlled substances as a patient for whom a licensed practitioner has prescribed them, when administering such drugs to patients on the order of a physician, or when acting as the official custodian of such drugs for an institution. Heavy penalties are imposed for the illegal possession of controlled drugs.

CANADIAN DRUG LEGISLATION

In Canada drug legislation exists to protect the consumer from fraud and deception in the sale and use of foods, drugs, cosmetics, and medical devices. The Food and Drug Directorate of the Department of National Health and Welfare is responsible for administration and enforcement of Canada's drug laws.

The present Canadian **Food and Drugs Act** was passed in 1953, amended in 1961 to provide greater control over barbiturates and amphetamines, and again in 1962 and 1969 to prohibit the sale of certain drugs. Major provisions of various schedules of the Act are as follows:

Schedule A. No food, drug, cosmetic, or device is to be advertised or sold as a treatment, preventative, or cure for certain listed diseases such as cancer and alcoholism.

Schedule B. Unless labeled otherwise, drugs must comply with standards prescribed in certain recognized pharmacopeias and formularies such as the U.S.P. and the British Pharmacopoeia.

Schedules C and D. Sale of listed drugs is prohibited unless the manufacturing process and premises have been approved by the Minister of National Health and Welfare.

Schedule E. Batch approval must be met before marketing of drugs listed. Sample distribution of drugs is prohibited except to physicians, dentists, and pharmacists.

Schedule F. No person shall sell any drug described in Schedule F, for example, thalidomide.

Schedule G. Controlled drugs are listed for which a license is required to import, manufacture, distribute, or dispense, and special records must be kept.

Schedule H. Restricted drugs are listed for which general use is prohibited because of high-abuse potential. This schedule compares with Schedule I, U.S. Controlled Substances Act.

The Canadian **Narcotic Control Act,** passed in 1961 with subsequent amendments, regulates the possession, sale, manufacture, production, and distribution of narcotic drugs.

Provincial laws also exist that modify the national laws governing the sale and administration of narcotics and dangerous drugs.

PROBLEMS

Name ______________________

Date ______________________

Consult your text and reference books to obtain the necessary information on standardization of drugs, drug standards, and legislation.

I. Standardization of drugs.

A. Methods by which drugs are standardized.

B. Method of preference.

II. Drug standards. The following titles indicate sources of information on drugs for pharmacists, physicians, and nurses. (1) By whom is each book compiled? (2) How often is each book revised? (3) Which of the books are legal standards?

A. The United States Pharmacopeia–National Formulary

B. United States Pharmacopeia Dispensing Information

C. The American Hospital Formulary Service

D. The Dispensatory of the United States of America

E. Physician's Desk Reference

III. Legislation. Give the objectives and provisions of the following Acts:

A. United States

1. Federal Food, Drug, and Cosmetics Act

Amendments:

a. Durham-Humphrey Amendment

b. Kefauver-Harris Amendment

c. Drug Abuse Control Amendment

2. Harrison Drug Act

Amendment:

a. Narcotic Control Act of 1956

3. Comprehensive Drug Abuse Prevention and Control Act of 1970

B. State

From your pharmacist or State Board of Pharmacy find out what laws your state has regarding the use and sale of habit-forming and harmful drugs.

C. Canada

1. The Food and Drugs Act

2. Canadian Narcotic Control Act

APPENDIX B

Common Arithmetic Terms

addend Any one of the numbers to be added in an addition problem.

approximate A "nearly correct" answer, not necessarily the exact answer.

common denominator A number that is evenly divisible by all the denominators of two or more fractions.

decimal An abbreviation for a fraction with a denominator of 10, 100, 1000, and so on. Only the numerator of the fraction is written. The location of the decimal point shows what the denominator is.

denominator The term below the fraction line in a fraction. It tells into how many parts a whole quantity is divided.

difference The answer to a problem in subtraction.

digit Any of the numerals 0, 1, 2, 3, 4, 5, 6, 7, 8, 9. The number 6789 has four digits: 6, 7, 8, 9.

dividend The number that is to be divided in a division problem.

divisor The number by which the dividend is divided in a division problem.

equivalent Equal to.

factor Any one of the numbers to be multiplied in a multiplication problem.

fraction A numeral representing the parts being considered out of a total number of parts in a whole quantity, for example, $1/5$ represents one of five equal parts of a whole quantity.

improper fraction A fraction in which the numerator is equal to or greater than the denominator.

integer A whole number.

invert To turn "upside down."

lowest common denominator The smallest number that is evenly divisible by the denominator of two or more fractions.

minuend The number from which another number is subtracted.

mixed number A number consisting of an integer (whole number) and a fraction.

multiplicand The number that is multiplied in a multiplication problem.

multiplier The number "multiplied by" in a multiplication problem.

numeral A name or symbol that represents a number.

numerator The part of a fraction that is above the line. It tells the number of parts of the divided unit that is being considered.

percent A fraction whose numerator is expressed and whose denominator is understood to be 100. The symbol % indicates percent.

product The answer to a multiplication problem.

proper fraction A fraction whose numerator is less than its denominator. Also called simple or common fraction.

proportion Consists of two ratios that are equal to each other.

quotient The answer to a division problem.

ratio The relationship of one quantity to another. It indicates division.

segment A part of a whole quantity.

subtrahend The number that is subtracted in a subtraction problem.

sum The result of simple addition.

symbol A letter or mark representing a number, a quantity, an operation, etc.

term Any of the parts composing a fraction, a proportion, or a ratio.

unit A whole quantity.

APPENDIX C

Tables of Abbreviations and Equivalents

Table of abbreviations for prescriptions and orders

Abbreviation	Meaning	Abbreviation	Meaning
aa	of each	o.h. or q.h.	every hour
a.c.	before meals	ol.	oil
ad.	up to	o.m.	every morning
ad lib.	as desired	o.n.	every night
aq.	water	os	mouth
aq. dest.	distilled water	O.S.	in left eye
b.i.d.	twice a day	O.U.	in each eye
c̄	with	oz. or ℥	ounce
caps.	capsules	p.c.	after meals
comp.	compound	per	by
dil.	dilute	pil.	pill
elix.	elixir	p.r.n.	when required
ext.	extract	q. 2 h.	every 2 hours
fld. or fl.	fluid	q. 3 h.	every 3 hours
Ft.	make	q. 4 h.	every 4 hours
g	gram	q.i.d.	four times a day
gr	grain	q.s.	quantity sufficient
gtt.	drop	℞	take
H.	by hypodermic	s	without
h.	hour	s.c.	subcutaneously
h.s.	hour of sleep	Sig.	write on label
I.M.	intramuscularly	sol.	solution
I.V.	intravenously	s.o.s.	once if necessary
M.	mix	sp.	spirits
♏ or m	minim	ss	one half
μg	microgram	stat.	immediately
mg	milligram	t.i.d.	three times a day
mixt.	mixture	tr.	tincture
ml	milliliter	U	unit
O	pint	ung.	ointment
O.D.	in right eye	vin.	wine
o.d. or q.d.	every day		

Table of metric doses with approximate apothecary equivalents

Metric	Approximate apothecary equivalents	Metric	Approximate apothecary equivalents
LIQUID MEASURE			
1000 ml	1 quart	3 ml	45 minims
750 ml	1½ pints	2 ml	30 minims
500 ml	1 pint	1 ml	15 minims
250 ml	8 fluid ounces	0.75 ml	12 minims
200 ml	7 fluid ounces	0.6 ml	10 minims
100 ml	3½ fluid ounces	0.5 ml	8 minims
50 ml	1¾ fluid ounces	0.3 ml	5 minims
30 ml	1 fluid ounce	0.25 ml	4 minims
15 ml	4 fluid drams	0.2 ml	3 minims
10 ml	2½ fluid drams	0.1 ml	1½ minims
8 ml	2 fluid drams	0.06 ml	1 minim
5 ml	1¼ fluid drams	0.05 ml	¾ minim
4 ml	1 fluid dram	0.03 ml	½ minim
WEIGHT			
30 g	1 ounce	30 mg	½ grain
15 g	4 drams	25 mg	⅜ grain
10 g	2½ drams	20 mg	⅓ grain
7.5 g	2 drams	15 mg	¼ grain
6 g	90 grains	12 mg	⅕ grain
5 g	75 grains	10 mg	⅙ grain
4 g	60 grains (1 dram)	8 mg	⅛ grain
3 g	45 grains	6 mg	1/10 grain
2 g	30 grains (½ dram)	5 mg	1/12 grain
1.5 g	22 grains	4 mg	1/15 grain
1 g	15 grains	3 mg	1/20 grain
0.75 g	12 grains	2 mg	1/30 grain
0.6 g	10 grains	1.5 mg	1/40 grain
0.5 g	7½ grains	1.2 mg	1/50 grain
0.4 g	6 grains	1 mg	1/60 grain
0.3 g	5 grains	0.8 mg	1/80 grain
0.25 g	4 grains	0.6 mg	1/100 grain
0.2 g	3 grains	0.5 mg	1/120 grain
0.15 g	2½ grains	0.4 mg	1/150 grain
0.12 g	2 grains	0.3 mg	1/200 grain
0.1 g	1½ grains	0.25 mg	1/250 grain
75 mg	1¼ grains	0.2 mg	1/300 grain
60 mg	1 grain	0.15 mg	1/400 grain
50 mg	¾ grain	0.12 mg	1/500 grain
40 mg	⅔ grain	0.1 mg	1/600 grain

Table of frequently used equivalents

		WEIGHT		
1 dram	=	60 grains	=	4 g
1 ounce	=	480 grains (8 drams)	=	30 g
1 milligram	=	1/60 grain	=	0.001 g
100 milligrams	=	1½ grains	=	0.1 g
1 gram	=	15 grains	=	0.001 kg
1 kilogram	=	2.2 pounds (avoirdupois)	=	1000 g
		LIQUID		
1 fluid dram	=	60 minims	=	4 ml
1 fluid ounce	=	8 fluid drams	=	30 ml
1 pint	=	16 fluid ounces	=	480 ml
1 quart	=	32 fluid ounces	=	1000 ml
1 gallon	=	128 fluid ounces	=	3800 ml
1 teaspoonful	=	1 fluid dram	=	4 or 5 ml
1 tablespoonful	=	½ fluid ounce	=	15 ml
1 teacupful	=	6 fluid ounces	=	180 ml
1 glassful	=	8 fluid ounces	=	240 ml
		LENGTH		
1 inch	=	25 millimeters	=	2.5 cm
1 foot	=	12 inches	=	30.5 cm
1 yard	=	36 inches	=	0.9 m
1 mile	=	5280 feet	=	1.6 km

APPENDIX D

Summary of Pediatric Dosage Rules

CLARK'S RULE

$$\text{child's dose} = \frac{\text{weight in pounds}}{150} \times \text{adult dose}$$

Use only for children under 2 years of age and only as a rough estimate. Generally, the younger the child, the less reliable the rule.

YOUNG'S RULE

$$\text{child's dose} = \frac{\text{age in years}}{\text{age in years} + 12} \times \text{adult dose}$$

Use only for children over 2 years of age and only as a rough estimate. Dosage based on age shows considerable variability because of weight differences in children of a given age.

FRIED'S RULE

$$\text{child's dose} = \frac{\text{age in months}}{150} \times \text{adult dose}$$

Use only for children under 2 years of age. Like Young's Rule, this calculation does not take the weight of the child into consideration.

SURFACE AREA METHOD

$$\text{child's dose} = \frac{\text{child's body surface in m}^2}{1.7} \times \text{adult dose}$$

This is the most accurate method of calculating a child's dose from an adult dose and can be used for all children except neonates. To arrive at the surface area, determine the height and weight of the child and refer to any surface area chart.

APPENDIX E

Name ______________________

Date ______________________

Survey Test

The first four chapters in the workbook deal with basic arithmetic and are presented as review material.

We suggest that the student receive the workbook several weeks before class instruction begins so that the first four chapters can be reviewed out of class in preparation for the survey test. After the test is scored, errors will direct the instructor and the student to the types of problems the student must learn to solve to have the basic arithmetic knowledge needed for the study of drugs and solutions.

CHAPTER 1

Express the following in Roman numerals:

1. 9 ____________
2. 56 ____________
3. 90 ____________
4. 510 ____________
5. 2500 ____________

CHAPTER 2

Match the items in Column 1 with the correct phrase in Column 2:

Column 1

1. In the fraction $\frac{3}{8}$, 8 represents ____
2. $\frac{3}{5}$ is ____
3. $2\frac{1}{2}$ is ____
4. $\frac{9}{6}$ is ____
5. $\frac{3/4}{1/2}$ is ____

Column 2

a. A complicated fraction
b. A complex fraction
c. A denominator
d. An improper fraction
e. A mixed number
f. A proper fraction
g. A numerator
h. A reciprocal

Find the answers to these problems:

6. $\frac{5}{9} + \frac{7}{9}$

7. $\frac{3}{8} + \frac{5}{6}$

8. $2\frac{7}{10} + 3\frac{7}{8} + 4\frac{4}{5}$

9. $8\frac{7}{12} - \frac{1}{3}$

10. $7\frac{1}{2} - 2\frac{2}{3}$

11. $5 - \frac{7}{8}$

12. $\frac{8}{9} \times \frac{3}{16}$

13. $2\frac{1}{2} \times 1\frac{1}{10}$

14. $\frac{2}{3} \times \frac{5}{7} \times \frac{2}{3}$

15. $\frac{2}{5} \div 4$

16. $4\frac{2}{5} \div 8$

17. $\frac{4}{5} \div 2\frac{2}{3}$

Change to improper fractions, mixed numbers, or whole numbers:

18. $3\frac{2}{3}$

19. $\frac{5}{2}$

20. $\frac{13}{4}$

21. $\frac{16}{8}$

Name ____________________

Date ____________________

SURVEY TEST—cont'd

For these exercises, find the answer or simplify:

22. $\frac{3}{8} \div \frac{1}{4}$

23. $\dfrac{7/8}{4}$

24. $\frac{1}{4}$ of $\frac{5}{8}$

25. $\dfrac{2/3}{3/4}$

26. $4:5::8:x$

27. $\frac{6}{32}$

CHAPTER 3

Express each as a common fraction and as a decimal fraction:

1. Three hundredths ____________; ____________
2. Seven ten thousandths ____________; ____________
3. Five and seven tenths ____________; ____________

Complete the following, writing the answer in the blank spaces:

4. Placing a zero **before** the decimal point in 2. ____________ its value ______ times.
5. Placing a zero **after** the decimal point in 0.2 ____________ its value ______ times.
6. Placing two zeros before the decimal point in 2. ____________ its value ______ times.

7. Moving the decimal point to the right one place ________________ the value of a number by ______.
8. Nine multiplied by zero equals ______.
9. The least value decimal fraction in this list is
   a. 0.06
   b. 0.6
   c. 0.006
   d. 6.05
   e. 0.6056
10. Place the decimal point in each product in the proper place.
   a. $0.04 \times 0.3968 = 15872$ b. $3.02 \times 2.93 = 88486$
11. Place the decimal point in each quotient correctly.
   a. $74\overline{)\,.225404}$ with quotient 3046   b. $0.74\overline{)\,225404}$ with quotient 3046

Find the answers to the following:

12. $25.75 + 2\frac{1}{2}$

13. $0.2 + 0.005 + 0.6023 + 0.44$

14. $5. + 3.7 \times 0.37$

15. $46.008 - 4.7$

16. $58.9 - 26.0056$

17. $31. - 11.55$

18. $4.5 - 0.045$

19. 0.53×0.02

20. 0.5×4

21. 1.45×0.005

Name ______________________

Date ______________________

SURVEY TEST—cont'd

Find the answers to the following—cont'd

22. $55 \div 5000$

23. $8 \div 0.5$

24. $4.2 \div 2.1$

25. $136.08 \div 5.6$

26. $9 \div 0.03$

27. $14.5 \div 0.1$

28. $14.5 \div 10$

29. $14.5 \div 0.001$

30. $10.68 \times 2\frac{1}{4}$

Express the following decimal fractions as common fractions and as ratios. Reduce to lowest terms or simplest form:

	Decimal fraction	Common fraction	Ratio
31.	0.5		
32.	0.01		
33.	0.25		
34.	0.50		
35.	0.2		

Change to decimal fractions. Carry to three decimal places:

36. $\frac{1}{8}$

39. $\frac{2}{9}$

37. $\frac{2}{3}$

40. $2\frac{3}{4}$

38. $1\frac{1}{12}$

CHAPTER 4

Match the items in Column 1 with the correct answers from Column 2. Identify the answer by their corresponding letters:

Column 1		Column 2	
1. $\frac{1}{2}$% ____		a. 0.0005	f. $\frac{1}{4}$
2. $6\frac{2}{3}$% ____		b. 0.015	g. $2\frac{1}{2}$
3. 25% ____		c. 0.75%	h. $\frac{100}{2}$
4. $0.00\frac{1}{2}$ ____		d. 75%	i. $\frac{20}{3}$
5. 0.0075 ____		e. $\frac{1}{15}$	j. $\frac{1}{200}$

What percent of:

6. 25 is 5?

8. 50 is 4?

7. 20 is 2?

Name ____________________

Date ____________________

SURVEY TEST—cont'd

Find percent:

9. 8% of 40?

10. $33\frac{1}{3}$% of 60?

11. $\frac{1}{2}$% of 450?

Find the value of x:

12. $3:5::x - 10:25$

13. $x + 1:12::6:10$

14. $0.01:10::x:4$

15. $\frac{1}{2}:50::x:200$

Convert the following:

16. Express $\frac{1}{8}$ as a percent. ____________

17. Change $\frac{1}{5}$% to decimal form. ____________

18. Change the ratio 1:100 to %. ____________

19. Change 0.2 to %. ____________

20. Change $2\frac{1}{8}$% to decimal form. ____________

21. Change 175% to a fraction. ____________

22. 3 = ______% of 9. ______

23. 125% of 60 = ______. ______

24. If 1.8 is 3% of a number, what is 100% of the number? ______

APPENDIX F

Name ____________

Date ____________

Comprehensive Examination for Review

Solve the following problems:

1. How much boric acid is needed to make 500 ml of 2% solution?

   ____

2. How many 0.2-g (gr iii) tablets are needed to make 240 ml of 2% solution?

   ____

3. How many milliliters of 1:750 benzalkonium chloride are needed to prepare 500 ml of 1:10,000 solution?

   ____

4. How many 0.5-g (gr viiss) tablets are needed to make 1 liter of 1:500 solution?

   ____

5. A solution containing 50,000 U of Polymyxin B sulfate in 250 ml is needed for an irrigating solution. The drug available is 250,000 U in 10 ml. How much drug will be used?

____

6. On hand is 4 ml of 2% cocaine solution. How much water must be added to make a ½% solution?

____

7. There are 1000 ml of 2% solution in a container. How much water must be added to make a ½% solution?

____

8. How many sodium chloride tablets 1 g (gr xv) are needed to make 1 liter of a 0.9% solution?

____

9. How many grains of gentian violet are needed to prepare 120 ml of a 1:5000 solution?

____

Name ____________________

Date ____________________

COMPREHENSIVE EXAMINATION FOR REVIEW—cont'd

10. A prescription order directs the pharmacist to add gr 4 of codeine to 6 fluid ounces of syrup with a codeine concentration of 10 mg/5 ml. What is the dose of codeine per 5 ml in the final preparation?

    ____

11. A patient takes 1 teaspoonful of phenobarbital elixir (400 mg/100 ml) four times a day. How much phenobarbital does the patient take per dose?

    ____

12. How much pure drug (crystals) is needed to make 120 ml of 3% iodine solution?

    ____

13. On hand are morphine solutions containing 8 mg (gr 1/8)/ml and 15 mg (gr 1/4)/ml. How many milliliters of each strength solution would you need for the following dosages?

    a. 4 mg (gr 1/15) ____________; ____________

    b. 10 mg (gr 1/6) ____________; ____________

    c. 30 mg (gr 1/2) ____________; ____________

    d. 6 mg (gr 1/10) ____________; ____________

14. On hand is 0.4 mg (gr $^{1}/_{150}$) atropine per milliliter. How many milliliters are needed to give the following?

a. 0.6 mg (gr $^{1}/_{100}$) ______________

b. 1.2 mg (gr $^{1}/_{50}$) ______________

c. 0.2 mg (gr $^{1}/_{300}$) ______________

d. 0.3 mg (gr $^{1}/_{200}$) ______________

15. On hand is 0.4 mg (gr $^{1}/_{150}$) scopolamine in 0.5 ml. How many milliliters are needed to give the following doses?

a. 0.3 mg (gr $^{1}/_{200}$) ______________

b. 0.8 mg (gr $^{1}/_{80}$) ______________

16. The adult dose of quinine is 0.3 g (gr v). (a) Compute the dosage for a 3-year-old child. (b) What law do you use?

a. ______________; b. ______________

17. The adult dose of Mandelamine as a urinary antiseptic is 0.5 g (gr $7\frac{1}{2}$). Compute the dosage for a 6-year-old child.

____

18. The adult dose of aspirin is 0.3 g (gr v). (a) Compute the dosage for a 10-month-old infant. (b) What law do you use?

a. ______________; b. ______________

Name ____________________

Date ____________________

COMPREHENSIVE EXAMINATION FOR REVIEW—cont'd

19. The adult dose of calcium lactate is 1 g (gr xv). Calculate the dosage for a 4-month-old infant.

 ____

20. The adult dose of a drug is 0.6 g (gr x). (a) Calculate the dose for a child weighing 70 pounds with a body surface area of 1.1 square meters. (b) Name the rule used.

 a. ____________; b. ____________

21. A stock vial of codeine sulfate is labeled gr xx in 20 ml. How much is needed to give the following?

 a. gr iss ____________

 b. gr 1/4 ____________

 c. gr ss ____________

 d. gr 3/4 ____________

22. A stock vial of morphine sulfate is labeled gr v in 20 ml. How much is needed to give the following?

 a. gr 1/4 ____________

 b. gr ss ____________

 c. gr 1/8 ____________

 d. gr 1/16 ____________

23. What is the amount of belladonna tincture per dose from the following prescription?

 ℞ Tr Belladonna fl ʒ iv
 Codeine phos gr vi
 Phenobarbital elix. q.s. ad. fl ℥ vi
 Sig: 1 tsp h.s.

24. A stock solution of Solu-Medrol is available containing 1000 mg in 16 ml. How much is needed to give 125 mg?

____

25. What is the ratio and percentage of the following solutions?

a. One-half liter containing 4 ml alcohol. ________; ________

b. 500 ml of glucose solution containing 25 g.

________; ________

c. 1 ml of solution containing 20 mg (gr ⅓). ________; ________

d. 100 ml containing ʒ i of drug. ________; ________

e. 100 ml of boric acid solution containing gr xv of drug.

________; ________

f. 24 ml of drug in 2000 ml solution. ________; ________

g. 20 ml of morphine sulfate solution containing 1.5 g.

________; ________

h. One liter containing 1 g of drug. ________; ________

Name ______________________

Date ______________________

COMPREHENSIVE EXAMINATION FOR REVIEW—cont'd

26. How many minims of insulin would be needed to give the following?

    a. U 35 of U 40 insulin ____________

    b. U 60 of U 100 insulin ____________

    c. U 80 of U 100 insulin ____________

    d. U 30 of U 100 insulin ____________

27. How many minims of penicillin solution will be needed to give the following?

    a. 300,000 U from a solution containing 500,000 U/ml. ____________

    b. 200,000 U from a solution containing 100,000 U/ml. ____________

    c. 80,000 U from a solution containing 100,000 U/ml. ____________

    d. 150,000 U from a solution containing 200,000 U/ml. ____________

    e. 25,000 U from a solution containing 40,000 U/ml. ____________

28. A 50-mg vial of sodium nitroprusside is added to 250 ml 5% dextrose solution. What is the concentration of the final solution in micrograms per milliliter?

____

29. Carbenicillin is ordered to be given intravenously in a dose of 400 mg/kg/day. The patient weighs 65 kg. How many grams/day need to be prepared?

____

30. Give 1 mg of Isuprel intravenously in 200 ml of 5% Dextrose over the next 3 hours. What is the infusion rate in drops per minute? (Standard Drop Factor of 10.)

____

31. How much lidocaine must be added to 250 ml 5% dextrose solution to obtain a final concentration of 4 mg/ml?

____

32. A vial of Bacitracin contains 50,000 units. How many milliliters should be added to the vial to prepare a solution containing 2500 units/ml?

____

Name ______________________

Date ______________________

COMPREHENSIVE EXAMINATION FOR REVIEW—cont'd

33. Cytomel 40 μg daily is ordered. Tablets available are 5 μg, 25 μg, and 50 μg. What tablets would you give for this dose?

    ____

34. How many mEq of $NaHCO_3$ (MW = 84) are contained in a 50-ml ampule of 8.4%?

    ____

35. How many ml of 19.6% potassium acetate (MW = 98.1) are needed to fill a hyperalimentation order for the addition of 30 mEq?

    ____

36. Changing Fahrenheit and Celsius temperature:

    a. 45° C to F ____________

    b. 149° F to C ____________

c. 96.8° F to C ______

d. 30° C to F ______

e. 104° F to C ______

f. 230° F to C ______

37. A 20-ml vial of Amicar contains 250 mg/ml. Prepare a dose of 2 g.

______

38. An 8-ml vial of Tagamet contains 1.2 g. Prepare 300 mg.

______

Name ____________________

Date ____________________

COMPREHENSIVE EXAMINATION FOR REVIEW—cont'd

39. An ampule of Cleocin contains 0.6 g/4 ml. Prepare 400 mg for I.V.

____

40. A 50-mg ampule of nitroglycerin is added to 500 ml 5% dextrose solution. If the infusion rate is set to deliver 6 ml/hr, how many micrograms of nitroglycerin will the patient receive per minute?

____

41. The usual dose of mithramycin used to treat hypercalcemia is 25 μg/kg. What dose would be required for a patient who weighs 150 pounds?

____

42. How long will it take for 1000 ml of 5% Dextrose in 0.2% Saline to be absorbed if the infusion rate is 30 gtt/min and the set has a Standard Drop Factor of 10?

____

43. When 95 ml of diluent is added to a 10-g vial of Geopen, a solution containing 1 g of Geopen per 10 ml is prepared. How much diluent should be added to a 10-g vial of Geopen to obtain a concentration of 1 g/5 ml?

____

44. The dosage requirement of an anticancer drug is 275 $mg/m^2/day$. The anticancer drug is available in a concentration of 200 mg/5 ml. What is the volume needed for a patient with a body surface area of 1.2 m^2?

____

45. The dose of Adriamycin to be given is 60 mg/m^2. The patient's body surface is 1.4 m^2. How many mg should be given?

____

46. An ampule of Intropin contains 200 mg/5 ml. The drug must be diluted before administration to the patient. How many ml of diluent must be used to give a final concentration of 800 $\mu g/ml$?

____

47. The children's dose of amoxicillin suspension is 40 mg/kg/day in divided doses every 8 hours. An 80-ml bottle contains 250 mg/5 ml. How many ml will you give for each dose to a child weighing 33 pounds?

____

Name ____________________

Date ____________________

COMPREHENSIVE EXAMINATION FOR REVIEW—cont'd

48. 1000 ml of 5% Dextrose in 0.45% Saline was started at 1:00 P.M. to be infused at 125 ml per hour. At 7:00 P.M. only 600 ml had been infused. Calculate the adjusted flow rate using a set with a Standard Drop Factor of 10.

____

49. Haldol concentrate contains 2 mg/ml. How many drops need to be given to administer a dose of 0.5 mg?

____

50. Corticotropin for injection has been reconstituted to provide 25 units/ml. (a) How much would you prepare for a dose of 20 units? (b) What type syringe would you use to administer this dose?

a. ____________; b. ____________

APPENDIX G

Answers to Problems

CHAPTER 1

Arabic and Roman number systems

p. 7.

1. LVI; C; XL; XXX; MDL; DCLVI; DIV; MCMLXXXV; CDXLVIII; LX; CCX; CMXIX; XXVII; LXXXV; XCIX; CCLIX
2. 250; 455; 1975; 94; 110; 29; 17; 33; 50; 95; 700; 650; 610; 2000; 4; 56; 9; 11; 1040; 89
3. vi; xiv; xxii; xix; mlxi; iii; li; vii; xviii; clv
4. 9; 24; 65; 4; 141; 40; 12; 29; 71; 35

CHAPTER 2

Fractions and ratio

p. 17. Changing to improper fractions

1. $\frac{17}{5}$
2. $\frac{62}{3}$
3. $\frac{100}{3}$
4. $\frac{27}{8}$
5. $\frac{67}{4}$
6. $\frac{8}{3}$

p. 17. Changing to mixed numbers

1. $8\frac{2}{3}$
2. $20\frac{3}{8}$
3. $44\frac{1}{4}$
4. $6\frac{1}{2}$
5. $13\frac{5}{7}$
6. $13\frac{4}{5}$

p. 17. Addition of fractions

1. $\frac{5}{6}$
2. $1\frac{17}{30}$
3. $1\frac{13}{24}$
4. $1\frac{20}{63}$
5. $15\frac{24}{27}$
6. $3\frac{4}{9}$

p. 18. Subtraction of fractions

1. $\frac{1}{9}$
2. $3\frac{1}{8}$
3. $2\frac{5}{16}$
4. $1\frac{1}{8}$
5. $\frac{8}{35}$
6. $\frac{9}{1000}$

pp. 18-19. Multiplication of fractions

1. $\frac{1}{9}$
2. $\frac{1}{10,000}$
3. $4\frac{1}{5}$
4. 4
5. $\frac{3}{16}$
6. $\frac{1}{16}$

p. 19. Division of fractions

1. $1\frac{1}{3}$
2. $\frac{1}{3}$
3. 26
4. $5\frac{1}{3}$
5. 10
6. 30

pp. 19-20. Changing to ratio in lowest terms

1. 1:8
2. 1:400
3. 1:10
4. 40:49
5. 1:2
6. $\frac{2}{3}$: $\frac{3}{8}$

p. 20. Changing to fractions in lowest terms

1. $\frac{1}{7}$
2. $\frac{1}{100}$
3. $\frac{3}{10}$
4. $\frac{1}{8}$
5. $\frac{1}{42}$
6. $\frac{1}{10}$

CHAPTER 3

Decimals

p. 22. Reading decimal numbers

1. Nine hundred seventy-eight and fifty-five hundredths
2. Nine and one-tenth
3. Two and five ten-thousandths
4. Forty-two and one one-thousandth or forty-two and one-thousandth
5. Forty-two and one ten-thousandth
6. Thirty-seven thousandths
7. Twenty-one hundredths
8. Eight thousand seven hundred fifty-six ten-thousandths
9. Nine-tenths
10. Fifteen thousand three hundred forty-one hundred-thousandths

p. 22. Determining the decimal fraction of the least value

1. 0.042
2. 0.0001
3. 0.3
4. 0.0007
5. 0.0022
6. 0.3
7. 0.25
8. 0.12

p. 24. Conversion of decimals to common fractions and ratio

1. $\frac{1}{4000}$; 1:4000
2. $\frac{1}{400}$; 1:400
3. $\frac{1}{3}$; 1:3
4. $\frac{1}{20}$; 1:20
5. $\frac{13}{200}$; 13:200
6. $\frac{101}{500}$; 101:500
7. $\frac{1}{40}$; 1:40
8. $\frac{209}{2000}$; 209:2000
9. $\frac{1}{100}$; 1:100
10. $\frac{1}{10}$; 1:10
11. $\frac{1}{1000}$; 1:1000
12. $\frac{11}{25}$; 11:25
13. $\frac{31}{40}$; 31:40
14. $\frac{23}{25}$; 23:25

p. 25. Addition of decimals

1. 642.988
2. 902.4042
3. 42.668
4. 1.035
5. 2361.0037
6. 45.7
7. 10.555
8. 706.4295
9. 5139.3
10. 2.384

pp. 25-26. Subtraction of decimals

1. 1946.05
2. 9.601
3. 0.75
4. 0.935
5. 195.15
6. 87.327
7. 1.825
8. 48.298
9. 0.818
10. 99.899

pp. 26-27. Multiplication of decimals

1. 1.5008
2. 290.736
3. 902.2255
4. 3.86353
5. 0.02625
6. 28.56
7. 32.5
8. 0.001875
9. 74529.
10. 0.00001

pp. 27-28. Division of decimals

1. 4432.
2. 37.08
3. 5.43
4. 280.
5. 333.33+
6. 0.726
7. 2.
8. 4.7
9. 140.97
10. 1420.

p. 28. Conversion to decimals

1. 0.625
2. 0.1
3. 0.001
4. 0.226
5. 0.12
6. 0.4285+
7. 0.0133+
8. 0.2
9. 0.002
10. 0.004

p. 29. Conversion of decimals to common fractions and ratio

1. $\frac{21}{200}$; 21:200
2. $\frac{1}{2}$; 1:2
3. $\frac{1}{20}$; 1:20
4. $\frac{1}{3}$; 1:3
5. $\frac{33}{100}$; 33:100
6. $\frac{11}{1250}$; 11:1250
7. $\frac{11}{20{,}000}$; 11:20,000
8. $\frac{7}{10}$; 7:10
9. $\frac{58}{125}$; 58:125
10. $\frac{9}{40}$; 9:40

CHAPTER 4

Percentage and proportion

p. 37. Changing percent to common fraction, decimal fraction, and ratio

1. $\frac{1}{2}$; 0.5; 1:2
2. $\frac{2}{3}$; $0.66\frac{2}{3}$; 2:3
3. $\frac{1}{3}$; $0.33\frac{1}{3}$; 1:3
4. $\frac{1}{40}$; 0.025; 1:40
5. $\frac{21}{400}$; 0.0525; 21:400
6. $\frac{11}{100}$; 0.11; 11:100
7. $\frac{12}{25}$; 0.48; 12:25
8. $\frac{23}{100}$; 0.23; 23:100
9. $\frac{3}{4}$; 0.75; 3:4
10. $\frac{3}{400}$; 0.0075; 3:400
11. $\frac{1}{1}$; 1.; 1:1
12. $\frac{1}{100}$; 0.01; 1:100
13. $\frac{1}{1000}$; 0.001; 1:1000
14. $\frac{1}{10}$; 0.001; 1:1000
15. $\frac{1}{40}$; 0.025; 1:40
16. $\frac{1}{4}$; 0.25; 1:4
17. $\frac{1}{400}$; 0.0025; 1:400
18. $\frac{37}{200}$; 0.185; 37:200
19. $\frac{19}{20}$; 0.95; 19:20
20. $\frac{29}{300}$; $0.0966\frac{2}{3}$; 29:300
21. $\frac{1}{25}$; 0.04; 1:25
22. $\frac{9}{200}$; 0.045; 9:200
23. $\frac{1}{800}$; 0.00125; 1:800
24. $\frac{3}{400}$; 0.0075; 3:400
25. $\frac{1}{250}$; 0.004; 1:250

pp. 37-38. Changing to percent

1. 30%
2. 75%
3. $212\frac{1}{2}$% or 212.5%
4. 0.1%
5. 1%
6. 0.1%
7. 1%
8. 350%
9. 57.7%
10. 25%
11. 1%
12. 50%
13. $0.33\frac{1}{3}$%
14. $83\frac{1}{3}$%

pp. 38-39. Finding what percent one number is of another

1. 5%
2. 55%
3. 33⅓%
4. 12%
5. 10%
6. 1%
7. 0.2%
8. 12.5%
9. 20%
10. 20%
11. 20%
12. 0.04%
13. 2%
14. 4%

pp. 39-40. Finding given percent of a number

1. 0.0525
2. 14.4
3. 2.25
4. 0.18
5. 416.25
6. 1.87½ or 1.875
7. 95
8. 0.7
9. 1.
10. 0.065625
11. 850.
12. 2205.
13. 58.8
14. 30.0

pp. 40-41. Finding the value of *x*

1. $x = 17$
2. $x = 5$
3. $x = 1000$
4. $x = 375$
5. $x = 10$
6. $x = 2001$; $x - 1 = 2000$
7. $x = 100$
8. $x = 800$
9. $x = 3/16$
10. $x = 540$
11. $x = 0.4$
12. $x = 121$; $x - 1 = 120$
13. $x = 500$
14. $x = 500$
15. $x = 15$
16. $x = 108$
17. $x = 12$
18. $x = 48$
19. $x = 63.75$
20. $x = 2$

pp. 42-44. Finding drug proportion

1. 1 oz, 6¼%
2. 40 oz
3. 3⅕ g or 3.2 g
4. 750 ml
5. 2000 ml
6. 25%
7. 0.2 ml
8. 3000 ml
9. 0.4 ml
10. 125,000 units
11. 50 mg
12. 5 ml
13. 18.9 ml
14. 11.3 g
15. 4.5 ml

CHAPTER 5

Apothecaries' system

pp. 49-50. Changing to equivalents within the system

1. fl ʒ ¼
2. fl ʒ 1
3. fl ℥ ½
4. ʒ ½
5. ℥ 2
6. ʒ ¼
7. fl ℥ 1
8. ♏ 30
9. fl ℥ 2; ♏ 960
10. fl ʒ 4; ♏ 240
11. qt 1; fl ʒ 256; ♏ 15,360
12. fl ʒ 6; ♏ 360
13. fl ʒ 8; fl ℥ 1
14. fl ʒ 2; fl ℥ ¼
15. pt 6; gal ¾
16. pt. 4; qts 2
17. fl ʒ 128; fl ℥ 16
18. fl ℥ 48; qt 1½; gal ⅜
19. lb. 1⅓
20. ʒ 20
21. lb. 1
22. ʒ 4; ℥ ½
23. ʒ 8; ℥ 1
24. ʒ 3; ℥ ⅜
25. ʒ 2; ℥ ¼

CHAPTER 6

Metric system

p. 55. Changing to equivalents within the system

1. 1 mg
2. 0.15 mg
3. 0.8 mg
4. 100 μg
5. 500 μg
6. 0.03 g
7. 0.004 g
8. 0.1 g
9. 0.01 g
10. 0.001 g
11. 0.85 g
12. 1.5 g

13. 6 mg
14. 65 mg
15. 1000 mg
16. 100 mg
17. 15,000 mg
18. 5000 mg
19. 500 mg
20. 250 mg
21. 1 kg
22. 0.1 kg
23. 1.5 kg
24. 500 g
25. 50 g
26. 8000 g
27. 0.5 l
28. 0.9 l
29. 100 ml
30. 1100 ml
31. 1000 ml
32. 7000 ml
33. 700 ml
34. 0.25 l
35. 0.675 l
36. 5 l

CHAPTER 7

System conversion and household equivalents

p. 61. Converting to units in the apothecaries' system

1. ♏ 60
2. ♏ 45
3. ♏ 5
4. ♏ 120
5. ♏ 30
6. fl ʒ 2
7. fl ʒ 3
8. fl ℥ 1
9. fl ʒ 6
10. pt 1
11. fl ℥ 10
12. fl ℥ 6
13. pt 1½
14. qt 2
15. gal 2½
16. qt 2½
17. gr 1/60
18. gr 1/600
19. gr 1/250
20. gr 1/120
21. ℥ 4
22. ʒ 1/1000
23. lb 2.2
24. lb 4.4
25. lb 1.1
26. gr 7½
27. gr 10
28. gr 5
29. gr ½
30. gr ½
31. gr 1
32. gr 1
33. gr 1½
34. gr 1½
35. gr 1/12
36. gr 1/60

p. 62. Converting to units in the metric system

1. 1 ml
2. 16 ml
3. 6 ml
4. 8 ml
5. 1⅔ ml
6. 60 mg
7. 0.065 g
8. 650 mg
9. 0.65 g
10. 2 g
11. 5 g
12. 120 mg
13. 12 mg
14. 0.6 mg
15. 10 g
16. 15 mg
17. 0.3 mg
18. 0.4 mg
19. 1 mg
20. 30 g
21. 100 g
22. 8 ml
23. 1 ml
24. 40 ml
25. 30 ml
26. 240 ml
27. 250 ml
28. 960 or 1000 ml
29. 6000 ml
30. 30 g
31. 30 g
32. 15 g
33. 360 g
34. 480 g
35. 300 g
36. 40 g

pp. 62-63. Changing to approximate equivalents in household measure

1. T ¼
2. gtts 60
3. fl ℥ ½
4. fl ℥ 4
5. fl ℥ 6
6. fl ℥ 2
7. fl ʒ 1
8. T 1
9. T 8
10. tsp 1
11. tsp 1½
12. tsp ½
13. T 4
14. pt 1
15. 2 glassfuls
16. 1 teacupful
17. 2 teaspoonfuls
18. T 2
19. tsp ⅓
20. 1 teacupful

CHAPTER 8

Temperature measurement

pp. 69-71. Converting from one temperature scale to the other

1. 122° F
2. 45° C
3. 100.4° F
4. 100° C
5. 32° F
6. 38° C
7. 20° C
8. 140° F
9. 59° F
10. 85° C
11. 22.2+ or 22 2/9° C
12. 20° C
13. a. 37° C
    b. 37.5+ or 37.6° C
14. 40° C
15. 104° F
16. 41° F
17. 48.8° C
18. 86° F
19. 4.4° C to 15.5° C
20. 35.6° F to 46.4° F

CHAPTER 9

Introduction to dosage

p. 81. Abbreviations

1. of each
2. before meals
3. ad.
4. ad lib.
5. aq.
6. distilled water
7. b.i.d.
8. c̄
9. capsules
10. compound

11. dil.
12. elix.
13. ext.
14. fluid
15. Ft.
16. g
17. gr
18. drop
19. by hypodermic
20. hour
21. h.s.
22. intramuscularly
23. intravenously
24. kilogram
25. mix
26. milligram
27. milliliter
28. m or ♏
29. mixt.
30. O
31. q.d.
32. q.h.
33. every morning
34. every night
35. mouth
36. oz
37. after meals
38. by
39. pill
40. p.r.n.
41. q. 2 h.
42. q. 3 h.
43. q. 4 h.
44. q. 6 h.
45. 4 times a day
46. quantity sufficient
47. take
48. s̄
49. subcutaneously
50. write on label
51. sol.
52. once if necessary
53. sp.
54. ss
55. stat.
56. 3 times a day
57. tincture
58. U
59. ointment
60. wine

pp. 82-85. Interpreting orders

1. Ampicillin capsules 0.5 g every 4 hours, by mouth.
2. Nitroglycerin gr $\frac{1}{150}$ sublingually (under tongue) immediately and when required.
3. Erythromycin 250-mg tablet 3 times a day.
4. Calcium gluconate gr $7\frac{1}{2}$ intramuscularly from an ampule labeled 0.5 g in 2 ml.
5. Synkayvite 10 mg every day, intramuscularly.
6. Apply lanolin ointment to lips as desired.
7. Dalmane 15 mg by mouth once if necessary.
8. Aspirin and calcium carbonate gr 5 of each immediately and when required.
9. Valium 5 mg by mouth immediately and twice a day.
10. Regular insulin units 10, one-half hour before meals.
11. Morphine sulfate gr $\frac{1}{4}$ every 4 hours by hypodermic.
12. Apply neomycin solution to wound every 2 hours for 12 hours.
13. Dilute 4 ml procaine solution with sufficient distilled water to make 6 ml.
14. Tetracaine $\frac{1}{2}$% drops 2 in left eye immediately.
15. Elixir terpin hydrate with codeine ʒ 1 by mouth every 4 hours and when required.
16. Thyroid gr 3 by mouth, every day.
17. Procaine penicillin 600,000 units intramuscularly twice a day.
18. Fluid extract of cascara sagrada ʒ 2 by mouth as needed.
19. Elixir Benadryl ʒ $1\frac{1}{2}$ by mouth every morning and every night.
20. Sodium phenobarbital gr 2 subcutaneously at once.
21. Dilute with water ♏ 15 of tincture opium and give by mouth before meals twice a day.
22. Ferrous sulfate 0.3 g 3 times a day by mouth with meals or after meals.
23. Lanoxin 0.125 mg twice a day.
24. One (1) drop of pilocarpine 1% in each eye every day in afternoon (P.M.).
25. Timoptic 0.25% one drop in right eye every 12 hours.
26. Restoril 15 mg at bedtime; may repeat once if necessary.
27. Cold cream and white petrolatum, 1 ounce each. Mix and make an ointment. Apply at bedtime.
28. Feldene capsule 20 mg every morning.
29. Isoptocarpine 2%, 1 drop in the left eye four times a day.
30. Furosemide 80 mg intravenously every 12 hours.
31. Tincture camphorated opium 5 ml, one to four times a day and when required.
32. Dilute 0.5 ml. Haldol Concentrate with $\frac{1}{2}$ ounce of wine.
33. Serax 15 mg by mouth three times a day.
34. Heparin 5000 units subcutaneously every day.
35. Amitriptyline 25 mg 1 hour after meals and at bedtime.

CHAPTER 10

External dosage

pp. 101-102. Determining solutions from pure or full-strength drugs

1. 1000 ml
2. ℥ 1
3. 500 ml
4. 700 ml
5. gr 5; 0.3 g
6. 400 ml
7. 100 ml
8. 500 ml
9. 9 g; tsp $2\frac{1}{4}$
10. 8 g; tsp 2

pp. 103-104. Determining solutions from stock solutions

1. 20 ml
2. 100 ml
3. 500 ml
4. ʒ 2; 7½ ml
5. 50 ml
6. 500 ml
7. 140 ml
8. 200 ml
9. 444.4 ml
10. 600 ml

pp. 105-106. Determining the percentage strength of solutions

1. a. 1.2% or 1⅕%
   b. 0.025%
   c. 20%
   d. 66⅔%
   e. 8%
   f. 3.5% or 3½%
   g. 10%
   h. 50%
   i. 160%
   j. 0.1% or ⅒%
2. 10%
3. 0.2% or ⅕%
4. 0.1%
5. 25%
6. 12½% or 12.5%
7. 0.01%
8. 0.5% or ½%
9. 7.5% or 7½%
10. 1.6% or 1⅗%

pp. 107-108. Determining the ratio strength of solutions

1. a. 3:20
   b. 7:10
   c. 0.9:100
   d. 5:4
   e. 1:1
   f. 3:25
   g. 1:3
   h. 3:100
   i. 0.1:100
   j. 0.1:25
2. 1:6
3. 0.1:15 or 1:150
4. 0.1:200 or 1:2000
5. 0.3:50 or 3:500
6. 0.1:160 or 1:1600
7. 1:600
8. 1:25
9. 1:1000
10. 3:100

CHAPTER 11

Oral dosage

pp. 115-117. Determining oral dosage from stock solutions

1. 4 ml; ʒ 1
2. gr ¾
3. 1.25 ml
4. 12 ml
5. 11¼ ml; ʒ 3
6. 5 ml
7. fl ʒ 1
8. 16 mg
9. 6 ml; ʒ 1½
10. 12.5 ml; ʒ 3⅛
11. a. 7 ml.
    b. 4 ml.
12. ʒ 1½
13. 0.25 ml
14. 3.25 ml
15. a. 2000 mg; 50 ml
    b. 500 mg; 12.5 ml

pp. 118-122. Determining oral dosage from tablets and capsules

1. a. 2 tablets
   b. 1 tablet
   c. 1 tablet
2. 2 tablets
3. 2 tablets
4. 3 capsules
5. 2 tablets
6. 2 tablets
7. a. 2 tablets
   b. 1 tablet
8. a. 5 mg
   b. 3 tablets
9. 2 tablets
10. 4 tablets
11. a. 10 mg
    b. 3 tablets
12. 2 tablets
13. a. 4.2 g. Give 4 g.
    b. 1.05 g. Give 1 g.
    c. 2.1 tablets. Give 2 tab.
14. 0.5 g.
15. 8 capsules
16. a. 2 capsules
    b. 4 capsules
17. a. 2 capsules
    b. 3 capsules
    c. 2 capsules
18. a. 250 mg
    b. 250 mg
19. 3 capsules
20. 1 tablet
21. ½ tablet
22. a. 5 mg
    b. 2½ tablets
23. a. 600 mg
    b. 300 mg
24. a. 3000 mg
    b. 500 mg
25. 7 tablets

CHAPTER 12

Parenteral dosage

p. 131. Laboratory problems (insulin)

3. a. ♏ 5
   b. ♏ 5
   c. ♏ 5
   d. ♏ 6
4. a. ♏ 4
   b. ♏ 4

pp. 141-149. Calculating parenteral dosage

1. a. 0.3 ml or 3/10 ml or ♏ 5
   b. 1 ml
2. a. 2 ml
   b. 1⅓ ml or ♏ 20
3. a. 1⅕ ml
   b. 1½ ml
4. a. 2.5 mg ampule; use ⅘ or ♏ 12
   b. 10 mg ampule; use ⅘ or ♏ 12
5. a. 1½ ml
   b. 1¼ ml
6. a. 1½ ml
   b. ½ ml
7. a. ♏ 12
   b. ♏ 7½; use ½ ml
8. a. ♏ 15 or 1 ml
   b. ♏ 10
   c. ♏ 7½; use ½ ml
9. a. ♏ 18
   b. 2 ml
10. a. 1¼ ml; use ♏ 20
    b. 1½ ml
11. a. 2 ml
    b. 1½ ml
12. 15 ml
13. 200 ml
14. ♏ 9
15. ♏ 30 or 2 ml
16. a. 3 ml
    b. 1 ml
17. ♏ 9
18. ♏ 8
19. 1 ml
20. 2 ml
21. 2.5 ml
22. ♏ 9
23. ♏ 25
24. a. 1½ ml
    b. 4 ml
25. ♏ 12
26. 5 ml
27. a. ♏ 18
    b. ♏ 24
    c. ♏ 12
    d. 9 ml
28. a. (1) 16.6 ml
       (2) 10 ml
    b. (1) 20 ml
       (2) 4 ml
29. 0.5 ml
30. 0.75 ml
31. 1.5 ml
32. 1 ml
33. 1 ml
34. 4 ml
35. 7.5 ml
36. 0.75 ml
37. 2 ml
38. 0.15 ml
39. ♏ 6
40. 1.67 ml

pp. 149-152. Measuring mEq, mM, and mOsm

1. a. 6.25 ml
   b. 9.4 ml
   c. 4.7 ml
   d. 3 ml
   e. 12.5 ml
2. a. 8 ml
   b. 20 ml
   c. 12 ml
   d. 15 ml
   e. 35 ml
3. a. 2 ml
   b. 4 ml
   c. 1.5 ml
   d. 3 ml
   e. 5 ml
4. a. 6.7 ml
   b. 5 ml
   c. 3.3 ml
   d. 13.3 ml
   e. 20 ml
5. a. 35.1 ml
   b. 46.8 ml
   c. 29.2 ml
   d. 14 ml
   e. 11.7 ml
6. 3 ml
7. 15 ml
8. 8 ml
9. 1 ml
10. 22.5 ml
11. 4.6 mEq
12. 74.9 g
13. 76.9 mEq
14. 204 mOsm
15. 1388.9 mOsm

pp. 153-154. Calculating flow rate

1. 27.8 or 28 drops/min
2. 21 drops/min
3. 16.7 or 17 drops/min
4. a. 83.3 or 83 ml/hr
   b. 13.8 or 14 drops/min
   c. 10.4 drops/min
5. 41.7 or 42 drops/min
6. 25 drops/min
7. 37.5 drops/min
8. 7.5 drops/min
9. 52.5 drops/min
10. 43.75 drops/min

CHAPTER 13

Pediatric dosage

pp. 159-166. Calculating pediatric dosage

1. a. 0.15 g
   b. 0.5 g
   c. 2 ml
   d. $6\frac{2}{3}$ ml; use 7 ml
2. a. 0.11 mg, use 0.1 mg
   b. 0.53 mg; use 0.5 mg
3. 50 mg
4. a. U. 480,000
   b. 1.6 ml
   c. ♏ 24
5. a. 20 mg, total dose
   b. 5 mg, single dose
6. a. 0.1 g or gr $1\frac{1}{2}$
   b. ♏ 20
7. gr $\frac{2}{3}$
8. 0.38 ml or ♏ 6
9. a. gr $\frac{5}{68}$; give gr $\frac{1}{15}$
   b. gr $1\frac{8}{17}$; give gr $1\frac{1}{2}$
10. a. 23.7 mg or 24 mg
    b. 71.2 mg or 71 mg
11. $4\frac{2}{7}$ mg; give 4 mg or gr $\frac{1}{15}$
12. 3 ml
13. 50 mg
14. a. 353 mg
    b. 176.5 mg
15. 0.25 g
16. a. 4 mg
    b. 3 mg
17. 0.35 mg
18. 31.8 mg
19. a. 8.8 mg
    b. 4.7 mg
20. 50 mg
21. 750 mg
22. 1 ml
23. 1.4 mg
24. 42 tablets
25. 100 mg

APPENDIX E

Answers for survey test

p. 183. Chapter 1

1. IX
2. LVI
3. XC
4. DX
5. MMD

pp. 183-185. Chapter 2

1. c
2. f
3. e
4. d
5. b
6. $\frac{12}{9}$ or $1\frac{3}{9}$ or $1\frac{1}{3}$
7. $\frac{29}{24}$ or $1\frac{5}{24}$
8. $11\frac{3}{8}$
9. $8\frac{3}{12}$ or $8\frac{1}{4}$
10. $4\frac{5}{6}$
11. $4\frac{1}{8}$
12. $\frac{1}{6}$
13. $2\frac{3}{4}$
14. $\frac{20}{63}$
15. $\frac{1}{10}$
16. $\frac{11}{20}$
17. $\frac{3}{10}$
18. $\frac{11}{3}$
19. $2\frac{1}{2}$
20. $3\frac{1}{4}$
21. 2
22. $\frac{3}{2}$ or $1\frac{1}{2}$
23. $\frac{7}{32}$
24. $\frac{5}{32}$
25. $\frac{8}{9}$
26. 10
27. $\frac{3}{16}$

pp. 185-188. Chapter 3

1. $\frac{3}{100}$; 0.03
2. $\frac{7}{10,000}$; 0.0007
3. $5\frac{7}{10}$; 5.7
4. increases or multiplies; 10
5. decreases or divides; 10
6. increases or multiplies; 100
7. increases or multiplies; 10
8. zero
9. c (or 0.006)
10. a. 0.015872
    b. 8.8486
11. a. 0.003046
    b. 304600.
12. 28.25
13. 1.2473

14. 9.07
15. 41.308
16. 32.8944
17. 19.45
18. 4.455
19. 0.0106
20. 2.0
21. 0.00725
22. 0.011
23. 16.
24. 2.
25. 24.3
26. 300
27. 145.
28. 1.45
29. 14,500
30. 24.03
31. $\frac{5}{10}$ or $\frac{1}{2}$; 1:2
32. $\frac{1}{100}$; 1:100
33. $\frac{1}{4}$; 1:4
34. $\frac{1}{2}$; 1:2
35. $\frac{1}{5}$; 1:5
36. 0.125
37. $0.666\frac{2}{3}$
38. $1.083\frac{1}{3}$
39. $0.222\frac{2}{9}$
40. 2.75

pp. 188-190. Chapter 4

1. j
2. e
3. f
4. j
5. c
6. 20%
7. 10%
8. 8%
9. 3.20
10. 20.
11. 2.25
12. $x = 25; \therefore x - 10 = 15$
13. $x = 6.2; \therefore x + 1 = 7.2$
14. 0.004 or $\frac{1}{250}$
15. 2.
16. $12\frac{1}{2}$%
17. 0.002
18. 1%
19. 20%
20. 0.02125
21. $1\frac{3}{4}$
22. $33\frac{1}{3}$%
23. 75
24. 60

APPENDIX F

Answers for comprehensive examination for review

pp. 191-203.

1. 10 g or ʒ $2\frac{1}{2}$
2. 24 tablets
3. 37.5 ml
4. 4 tablets
5. 2 ml
6. ʒ 3 or 12 ml
7. 3000 ml or 3 qt
8. 9 tablets
9. gr 0.37
10. 17.2 mg/5 ml
11. 20 mg
12. 3.6 g; use ʒ 1
13. a. 0.5 ml; 0.27 ml
    b. 1.25 ml; 0.67 ml
    c. 3.75 ml; 2 ml
    d. 0.75 ml; 0.4 ml
14. a. 1.5 ml
    b. 3 ml
    c. 0.5 ml
    d. 0.75 ml
15. a. 0.38 ml
    b. 1 ml
16. a. gr 1 or 0.06 g
    b. Young's rule
17. 0.17 g or gr $2\frac{1}{2}$
18. a. gr $\frac{1}{3}$ or 0.02 g
    b. Fried's rule
19. gr $\frac{2}{5}$ or 0.026 g
20. a. 0.4 g or gr $6\frac{1}{2}$
    b. Surface area rule
    or
    a. 0.39 or gr 5
    b. Clark's rule (less accurate)
21. a. $1\frac{1}{2}$ ml
    b. $\frac{1}{4}$ ml or ♏ 4
    c. $\frac{1}{2}$ ml or ♏ 8
    d. $\frac{3}{4}$ ml or ♏ 12

22. a. 1 ml
    b. 2 ml
    c. ½ ml or ♏ 8
    d. ¼ ml or ♏ 4
23. 0.4 ml
24. 2 ml
25. a. 1:125; 0.8%
    b. 1:20; 5%
    c. 1:50; 2%
    d. 1:25; 4%
    e. 1:100; 1%
    f. 3:250; 1.2%
    g. 3:40; 7.5%
    h. 1:1000; 0.1%
26. a. ♏ 13
    b. ♏ 10
    c. ♏ 12
    d. ♏ 5
27. a. ♏ 9
    b. ♏ 32
    c. ♏ 12
    d. ♏ 12
    e. ♏ 10
28. 200 μg/ml
29. 26 g
30. 11 drops/min
31. 1 g
32. 20 ml
33. Eight 5-μg tablets
34. 50 mEq
35. 15 ml
36. a. 113° F
    b. 65° C
    c. 36° C
    d. 86° F
    e. 40° C
    f. 110° C
37. 8 ml
38. 2 ml
39. 2.67 ml
40. 10 μ
41. 1.7 mg
42. 5½ hr
43. 45 ml
44. 8.25 ml
45. 84 mg
46. 250 ml
47. 4 ml
48. 33.3 gtt/min
49. 4 gtt
50. a. 0.8 ml
    b. tuberculin

References

American Medical Association Department of Drugs: AMA drug evaluations, ed. 4, Littleton, Mass., 1983, Publishing Sciences Group Inc.

Baker, C. E., editor: Physicians' desk reference, ed. 36, Oradell, N.J., 1982, Medical Economics Co.

Cunningham, J. B.: Teaching metrics, Englewood Cliffs, N.J., 1976, Prentice-Hall, Inc.

Davis, N. M., and Cohen, M.: Medication errors: causes and prevention, Philadelphia, 1981, George F. Stickley.

Goodman, L. S., and Gilman, A., editors: The pharmacological basis of therapeutics, ed. 6, New York, 1980, The Macmillan Co.

Hahn, A. B., Barkin, R. L., and Oestreich, S. J. K.: Pharmacology in nursing, ed. 15, St. Louis, 1982, The C. V. Mosby Co.

Osol, A., and others, editors: Remington's pharmaceutical sciences, ed. 16, Easton, Pa., 1980, Mack Printing Co.

Shirkey, H. C., editor: Pediatric therapy, ed. 6, St. Louis, 1980, The C. V. Mosby Co.

The U.S. Pharmacoepia XX–National Formulary XV, Easton, Pa., 1980, Mack Publishing Co.